Advance Praise for
What, How Much & How to Eat

'In a sea of social media food myths, this book brings nutrition back to common sense rooted in Indian food. Clear, practical and empowering, it helps you understand what to eat without fear, fads or confusion.'

Dr Tanaya Narendra, author of *Dr Cuterus: Everything Nobody Tells You About Your Body*

'In a world filled with overconfident pseudoscience amplified by sensation-seeking algorithms, this book is a smart, evidence-based and practical guide that every Indian household will benefit from.'

Krish Ashok, author of *Masala Lab: The Science of Indian Cooking*

'Simple, doable, and refreshing – it shows you how to nourish yourself with ease, minus the stress.'

Rachana Ranade, finance educator

AF528910

What, How Much & How to Eat

What, How Much & How to Eat

Simple & Sustainable

Amita Gadre

BLOOMSBURY
NEW DELHI • LONDON • OXFORD • NEW YORK • SYDNEY

BLOOMSBURY INDIA
Bloomsbury Publishing India Pvt. Ltd
Second Floor, LSC Building No. 4, DDA Complex, Pocket C – 6 & 7,
Vasant Kunj, New Delhi, 110070

BLOOMSBURY, BLOOMSBURY INDIA and the Diana logo
are trademarks of Bloomsbury Publishing Plc

First published in India 2026

Copyright © Amita Gadre, 2026

Amita Gadre has asserted her moral rights to be identified as the author
of this work in accordance with the Indian Copyright Act, 1957

This book is not a substitute for medical attention, treatment, examination, advice, treatment of existing conditions or diagnosis. It is not intended to provide a clinical diagnosis nor take the place of medical advice from a fully qualified medical practitioner. Consult your healthcare service provider before following any health advice given in this book

All rights reserved. No part of this publication may be: i) reproduced or transmitted in any form, electronic or mechanical, including photocopying, recording or by means of any information storage or retrieval system without prior permission in writing from the publishers; or ii) used or reproduced in any way for the training, development or operation of artificial intelligence (AI) technologies, including generative AI technologies. The rights holders expressly reserve this publication from the text and data mining exception as per Article 4(3) of the Digital Single Market Directive (EU) 2019/790

ISBN: PB: 978-93-69528-50-9; eBook: 978-93-69527-71-7

2 4 6 8 10 9 7 5 3 1

Typeset in Bembo by Manipal Technologies Limited
Printed and bound in India by Thomson Press India Private Limited

FSC
www.fsc.org
MIX
Paper | Supporting responsible forestry
FSC® C010615

To find out more about our authors and books visit www.bloomsbury.com and sign up for our newsletters

Contents

For Raajas, may you always know food as nourishment, not confusion, and may eating be simple, joyful and free from fear

Introduction

Is a book on this topic really necessary? You would think not. In the current digital age, we are absolutely saturated with health, nutrition and wellness content every single time we open a social media app like Instagram, or even just browse the internet. With so much information available at our fingertips, one might assume the problem of knowledge has been solved.

But here is the twist: five years ago, I started making nutrition content on social media. Initially I used to speak about topics like 'how to lose weight sustainably', 'how to manage diet for diabetes', and so on. I later realised that the questions that plagued people the most were much simpler. Two years ago, as an extension of my short-form content on Instagram and Facebook, I started my own podcast dedicated entirely to the subject of nutrition. The response that the podcast received—the deluge of comments, questions and feedback—made me realise that people were not suffering from a simple lack of information; in fact, the opposite was true. They were suffering from a devastating abundance of misinformation—conflicting advice, sensationalised headlines, and diet myths that circulated relentlessly. And yes, the effect of this misinformation is actually devastating for many![1,2,3]

Most of the questions that people were asking seemed utterly straightforward, simple and fundamental to me, being trained and having practised as a nutritionist for years. But I know that they can be confusing, frustrating and even paralysing for the general public.

Let's look at the complexity of these common, real-world questions that flood my inbox and social media comments:

- **Protein Sources:** Are peanuts truly a good source of protein, or are they just a source of fat?
- **Dairy Consumption:** Do I need to consume milk as an adult, and does the type of milk matter?
- **The Ghar-ka-Khana Paradox:** Why are blood sugar levels inexplicably shooting up even when we are diligently eating regular, traditional, simple ghar ka khana (home-cooked food)?
- **The Ancestral Diet Dilemma:** Our parents and grandparents consumed plenty of ghee and oil, and seemingly did just fine, living long, healthy lives. So why are *we* as a generation struggling acutely with widespread health issues, obesity and chronic diseases now?
- **Hydration Timing:** What is the optimal time of day to drink water? Is it advisable or detrimental to drink water during meals?
- **The Multivitamin Mystery:** Why do we continue to experience persistent vitamin D deficiency even after taking expensive multivitamins or supplements regularly?
- **Carbohydrates and Weight:** Does eating rice, a staple of the Indian diet, inevitably lead to weight gain?
- **Home Remedies:** Can the practice of drinking bitter gourd or karela juice truly lower blood sugar levels, and is it safe to do so daily?

- **Cholesterol Fears:** Will consuming eggs, even just a few times a week, significantly increase my blood cholesterol levels?

I consistently dedicated all my content across social media to answering these 'simple' yet profoundly confusing questions, and the episodes reached lakhs of people across the country. That overwhelming, enthusiastic response made one thing clear—what feels obvious to a nutrition expert is still deeply confusing to a majority of people.

That realisation—that gap between expert knowledge and public understanding—is what pushed me to start writing this book. My hope is that this book will serve as a ready reference, offering clear, evidence-based insights about diet, food and nutrition. The overarching goal is not to put you on another restrictive, unsustainable diet but to empower you with a foundational understanding so robust that you can manage your daily diet confidently, and without falling prey to the endless, often dangerous, diet trends, fads and sensational claims that constantly circulate around you.

Once you have this basic knowledge, you will be able to decide for yourself, with critical thinking, whether those trends are actually helpful and scientifically sound, or merely marketing hype. You will be equipped to make truly informed, scientific and personalised decisions about your own plate. Most importantly, I will also take the time to explain the rationale behind the advice nutrition experts give, so you can understand *why* they make certain recommendations instead of just blindly following instructions.

This approach is deeply personal to me. As a child, I would always need to understand the reasons behind any advice given to me. Once I truly grasped the 'why', following the advice became straightforward and easy. Simply being told by adults 'because I said so' was never a satisfactory explanation for me. In my clinical practice today, I make it a central point to explain to all my patients exactly why certain nutritious foods are included in their custom diet plan, and why others are left out. I have consistently found that when patients understand the scientific reasoning and the *purpose* behind these choices, they develop a sense of ownership, and are far more likely to adhere to the guidelines and, as a result, achieve excellent, lasting health outcomes.

And that is exactly what we are going to do together in this book. We are going to explore not just the practical 'what to eat' and 'how much', but also understand the powerful, liberating *WHY!*

Let's start with **protein.**

I

Protein Is like God!

I am not about to break into a sermon here. What I truly mean to convey is that protein is, metaphorically, the God of our body—an omnipresent and foundational entity.

It is not merely a nutrient; it is the building block and the operational manager of our biological existence. Protein is an indispensable part of practically every action, every organ, and even the seemingly insignificant byproducts of our biology, like our sweat.

Here are all the places we find protein in our body: Protein forms the structural scaffolding of our cells, tissues and muscles. It exists as enzymes, powering the thousands of biochemical reactions necessary to keep us alive—from digesting the food we eat, to synthesising DNA. It is in our hormones, acting as messengers to coordinate complex bodily functions. It's in our blood, both as hemoglobin carrying life-giving oxygen, and as antibodies, our immune system's warriors.

Protein is the very essence of you. It is so fundamental to our being that one could literally imagine our body belting out a chartbuster like 'Hum tere bin ab reh nahi sakte, tere bina kya wajood mera' (I cannot live without you now, what is my existence without you) in the emotionally charged style of Arijit Singh, but with the song being a declaration of love and absolute dependency on PROTEIN.

So, what exactly is protein? Protein is literally the building block of every tissue, organ, cell in our body. Think of protein as the bricks that build our body's structural walls—inside as well as outside. Without these bricks, even the finest cement, paint or decorations (like vitamins and minerals) are useless. It's like painting a nonexistent wall; without protein, there's no foundation to support everything else.

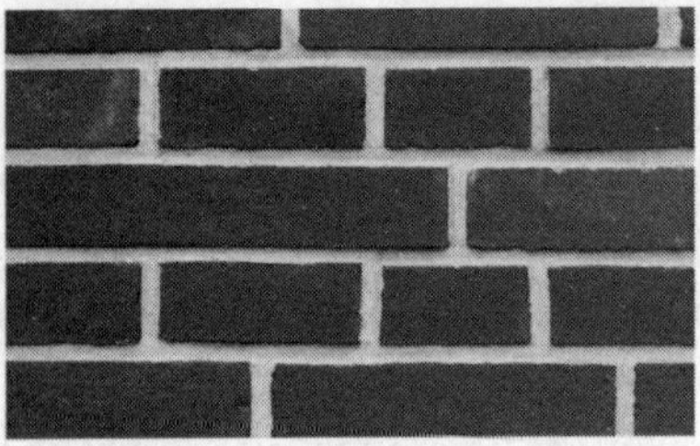

Image 1.1: *Protein as bricks in a wall*

If you've been scrolling through pages of fitness and wellness folks on Instagram lately, you probably already know that protein is a big deal in a healthy diet. But the minute I, as a nutritionist, suggest upping your protein, I get the same eye-roll reaction: 'Oh, great, here we go again—another wellness guru pushing those expensive, chemical-filled products from some pharma or supplement company.' This immediate leap to thinking that a high-protein diet requires protein powders, shakes or bars is a huge myth, and I'm here to bust it.

The simple truth? Getting enough protein absolutely does not mean you have to rely on supplements. In fact, our own traditional Indian food is perfectly capable of giving us all the protein we need, as long as we eat it in the right proportion and with a little thought.

The real problem isn't that our food lacks protein sources; it's that our non-stop, busy lives have messed up those traditional eating habits. This modern hustle often forces us to slap together incomplete, minimalist meals. Think about the Indian thali: dal/sambar, rice, roti, sabji, maybe some sprouts, and a salad. Preparing and eating that kind of variety every day has become a logistical nightmare for most people. Half of us don't know how to cook all of this, and the other half don't have the time.

No wonder then that when I tell people to eat a complete meal, I am always asked, 'Amita, with my crazy workday, how many lunchboxes are you realistically expecting me to carry?'

The result is that we often compromise, just packing roti and sabji, or a simple dal and rice for lunch. These meals are 'convenient' but incomplete.

Let's look at the numbers. In Indian cooking, our main protein stars are dals (pulses/lentils), various sprouts, and dairy like paneer and dahi or yogurt. For those who are non-vegetarian, meat, chicken, fish and eggs are excellent options.

Take the super common simple lunch: roti and sabji. In this meal, you'll get a measly 2 to 3 grams of protein at best, and most of that tiny amount actually comes from the wheat roti itself, not the veggies.

If you go for dal and rice, your protein intake does go up, but only slightly. You might get around 3 to 4 grams of protein from the dal. This number stays low for two main reasons. First, the dal in most homes or canteens is often watery; and second, hardly anyone consumes the two to three cups of dal needed to actually make a dent in their daily protein target in one sitting.

The main takeaway here is that yes, our traditional foods have protein, but our modern eating habits have left our typical meals protein-poor. The solution is in understanding the nutrition basics and planning our meals and meal choices with a healthful intent.

Here's a fact: Protein synthesis cannot happen on its own. Since protein is vital, we need to get it from our diet. Typically, we require about 0.8–1 gram[1] protein per kilogram of our ideal body weight. For instance, if your ideal weight is 60 kilograms, you should aim to consume around 60 grams of protein each day. If we have poha for breakfast (1 gram of protein), chapati and vegetable curry for lunch (2 grams of protein), vada pav with tea (2 grams of protein), and dal and rice for dinner (3 grams of protein), even with our best efforts, we would only manage to consume about 8–10 grams of protein in a day. That would be a daily protein deficit of 50 grams at the very least!

Food Item	**Protein (in grams)**
Pohe (Breakfast)	1 gram
Roti and vegetable curry (Lunch)	2 grams
Vada Pav (with Tea)	2 grams
(Thin) Dal Rice (Dinner)	3 grams
Total Protein	**8–10 grams**

Table 1.1: *The diet of a typical person throughout the day*

No surprises then that 'hair fall or hair loss' is a cosmetic or health problem on the rise! One of the primary reasons for hair loss is protein deficiency. But the first thing we think of when we start seeing hair fall or loss is biotin or multivitamins, because that's what is marketed to us! How will those B-complex vitamins work when you don't have the foundation of what actually makes your hair (keratin): protein!

A chronic protein deficiency will also make you feel weak, exhausted and cranky; it will make you feel low or encounter menstrual problems. And yet, when faced with these issues, people first think of 'sugary fruit juices' to get more energy, or sugary energy drinks or multivitamin capsules. But no one thinks of the protein!

> You might have heard of this…
>
> One gram of protein per kilogram of ideal body weight is a common recommendation. For instance, if a man weighs 70 kilograms, he should aim for 70 grams of protein. Likewise, a woman weighing 60 kilograms would need about 60 grams of protein. However, if someone weighs around 120 kilograms (overweight), they should not consume 120 grams of protein.[2]
>
> On the other hand, if your weight is 45 kilograms, you may need to increase your protein intake to support weight gain. I will explain how to determine these protein requirements further ahead.[3]

As a young nutrition graduate, when I started discussing protein, my aai would ask, 'I am 40 years old now, and I have been eating food for so many years, surely there must be some protein stored in my body, right? Can't my body tap into that store for protein? Why are you telling me that I have to eat protein every day?' That's a valid question!

The protein reserve in our bodies primarily comes from our muscles. We Indians are genetically predisposed to having a higher percentage of (abdominal) fat and a minimum percentage of muscle mass.[4] That's because most of us don't do any of the muscle maintenance activities like eating enough protein through our diet and exercising regularly, particularly strength training.

The **protein leverage hypothesis** explains why we often keep eating beyond what our body actually needs.[5] In simple terms, your body experiences a strong drive to meet its daily protein requirements. Until those needs are met, your brain keeps sending hunger signals, pushing you to eat. But we interpret those signals as 'I need to snack'. It is important to note here that it is highly likely that we would have already eaten enough carbs and fats. But because our body is sensitive to our protein requirements, it tells us to eat, hoping that we will end up eating *something* to meet that protein requirement. When your meals are short on protein, this biological 'hunger alarm' doesn't switch off, leading to excess calorie intake due to misinterpretation. Over time, this leads to weight gain. On the other hand, when your diet consistently includes adequate protein, your appetite naturally stabilises. You feel full sooner, your cravings drop and your overall food intake becomes more balanced.

The practical takeaway is simple: make sure every meal has a protein anchor, such as dal, beans, curd, paneer, eggs, fish or meat. Think of meeting your protein needs like switching off the hunger alarm; once it's silenced, your body can finally rest easy instead of demanding more food.

Muscles aren't just about biceps; every organ in our body consists of muscle, all our vital organs like heart, lungs, liver, uterus, stomach, kidney—everything is muscle tissue.

If we go for a long time without enough protein in our diet, we might first notice some common symptoms like weakness, trouble concentrating, constant hunger, sunken eyes, low hemoglobin levels, low blood pressure, frequent illnesses and hair loss. If we overlook these signs, the situation can escalate to muscle wasting. Protein is primarily stored in our muscles, and when the body lacks sufficient protein, it begins to weaken those muscles and utilise the amino acids from them to fulfill daily protein needs.

Let's understand a common problem with popular weight loss methods using this information. A common practice in weight loss diets is skipping meals. Those who are trying to lose weight often skip breakfast or dinner, or eat very, very little during their other three meals, hoping that it would help them lose weight 'quickly'. Most of the people trying this want to lose 'belly fat'. Misled by this notion of eating as few calories as possible, they adopt a diet consisting solely of boiled vegetables, soups and salads, which are low in protein and calories. These folks do end up losing a bit of weight on the weighing scale, *but* their belly fat remains pretty much intact, and their waist circumference does not change. In fact, the lack of protein causes their limbs to weaken, resulting in muscle loss, which makes their arms and legs appear thinner and their belly seem even larger. Why does this happen? Their belly and waist circumference increased due to fat accumulation over time. In their quest for weight loss, these patients severely restrict their diet, leading to a reduction in muscle mass, while the fat remains unchanged. A decrease in muscle mass translates to muscle weakness.[6] Furthermore, if you have diabetes, heart disease or cholesterol problems, and your doctor has recommended weight loss, but your belly circumference isn't budging, your heart health risk remains unchanged.[7] Ironically, the weight loss diet which one had embarked upon to get 'healthy' ends up weakening previously healthy muscles. Weak muscles, combined with the persistence of abdominal and visceral fat, eventually heighten the risk to your heart!

The primary goal of health efforts should not be weight loss at the expense of muscle mass, as this is detrimental in the long term. It is important to remember that muscle is not confined to our limbs; it is integral to our entire body, making up vital organs such as the heart, liver, kidneys, lungs and the intestines. When we adopt crash diets or suffer from protein deficiency, these essential organ muscles also weaken. Paradoxically, an extreme, protein-deficient weight loss diet can lead to a *net* weakening of vital organs. Therefore, the true measure of health involves managing body fat (which includes fat loss for those who are overweight), maintaining and strengthening muscle and bone mass, and ensuring good cardiovascular fitness (the ability to perform a stress test without excessive breathlessness).

Benefits of Protein

- **Staying full for longer:** Protein reduces cravings. It takes time to digest, which makes you feel fuller for longer, so you don't feel hungry as often.
- **Muscle building and fat burning:** Protein is essential for muscle growth. Muscles burn more calories, which helps reduce fat.
- **Appetite control:** A protein-rich diet helps you feel satiated for a longer time, preventing overeating.
- **Stabilising blood glucose levels:** Protein helps stabilise blood sugar levels, reducing the glycemic load and preventing sudden spikes in sugar.
- **Healthy hair:** Protein is also important for hair growth. Hair is made up of a protein called keratin.
- **Increased IQ in children:** It is essential for children to have enough protein in their diet for proper growth and development.

- **Glowing skin:** Protein is vital for the skin, helping it look fresh and healthy.
- **Boosting immunity:** Protein is crucial for our immune system. If we consume enough protein, it also helps enhance the efficacy of medications.
- **Reducing fatigue:** Many of my clients have shared that whenever they consume protein, they automatically feel more energetic. Their focus improves, and they do not experience fatigue.
- **Wound healing:** Protein plays an essential role in the healing process of wounds and other physical injuries.

Bottom line: If you want to improve your overall health, it is essential to consume enough protein.

How can you tell if you're eating enough protein?

In today's world, figuring this out has become much simpler, thanks to smartphones. While not perfectly precise, apps like MyFitnessPal, Noom or Calorie Tracker can offer a good estimate of your daily protein intake.

For those situations that call for exact figures, nutritionists use detailed food composition tables. However, for the purposes of general healthy eating, this level of detail is usually unnecessary.

Personally, I don't calculate my precise protein intake every day, nor do I obsessively try to hit, say, 60 grams daily. Instead, I maintain a good general awareness of the protein I've consumed throughout the day.

The real issue arises when protein is completely ignored. For example, making a meal solely out of roti and a small amount of sabzi, or grabbing a vada pav. This extreme lack of attention to protein is definitely not advisable from a health standpoint.

A 2017 survey by the Indian Market Research Bureau (IMRB) highlighted a critical issue: a significant 73 per cent of Indians were protein-deficient. Moreover, an alarming 93 per cent were unaware of how much protein they should be consuming daily. This widespread protein deficiency is particularly notable within the typical Indian diet, which is mostly rich in carbohydrate and fat, while grossly lacking in meeting even the most basic protein requirement.

Five popular foods that people think are high in protein but actually aren't!

1. Mushrooms: They barely have 2–3 grams of protein per 100 grams. They are great for fibre, but don't count them as a protein source.
2. Peanut butter: It packs more fat than protein.
3. Almond milk: It has just about a gram of protein per cup, compared to cow's milk, which has 7 grams.
4. Quinoa: It is a whole grain; it is primarily a carb. It needs to be paired with a proper protein source.
5. Broccoli: The protein content is far too little to make a difference.

A common misconception is that protein is primarily available only in non-vegetarian sources like fish, eggs, chicken and meat.

The truth is that we can also obtain protein from dairy products like milk, yogurt and cheese. Additionally, vegetarian protein sources such as sprouts, lentils and soy products like tofu, tempeh and soy chunks are excellent alternatives.

Our Protein Requirements

We need about 0.8–1 grams of protein per kilogram of body weight.[8] If your weight is between 60 and 70 kilograms, you will need to eat anywhere between 48 and 70 grams of protein as per this protein intake calculation. For most people, it is advisable to park your protein intake at 1 gram per kilograms of body weight. So, a person with an ideal body weight of 60 kilograms should be aiming to eat at least 60 grams of protein per day. I recommend aiming for the higher end of the range because, as you will see in the chapter ahead, it is not very easy to meet your protein requirements if you are not mindful of the presence of protein-rich foods in every meal. Also, when it comes to protein, it is better to keep a reasonable buffer than a deficit.

The protein requirement of 1 gram per kilogram (g/kg) of body weight is specifically based on a person's **ideal** body weight for their height, not their actual weight if they are overweight and sedentary.

For an overweight person, using their actual weight would lead to an excessively high protein intake, potentially hindering weight loss. For instance, a person weighing 120 kilograms would consume 120 grams of protein daily using the 1g/kg calculation. However, if their ideal weight is closer to 65–70 kilograms, this high protein consumption (120 g) would likely result in an excess of total daily calories, ultimately causing weight gain rather than the desired weight loss.

It is also important to remember here that protein-rich foods also contain fat (for non-vegetarian sources) and carbs (for vegetarian sources). So, when planning a meal for an overweight person and planning their protein intake, we also need to take into account the other macronutrients that come with the protein-rich food—namely fat and carbs.

The recommended daily protein intake is **0.8 to 1.0 gram per kilogram of ideal body weight**.

This recommendation should be adjusted based on your goals:

- **For weight loss:** Aim for **0.8 gram of protein per kilogram of your** ideal **body weight**. For example, if your current weight is 120 kilograms but your ideal weight based on height is 65 kilograms,[9] you should calculate your protein needs based on 65 kilograms (65 multiplied by 0.8).
- **For building muscle and increasing lean mass:** Consume **1.0 to 1.2 grams of protein per kilogram of your** current **weight**. This range depends on your workout intensity and the amount of weight you intend to gain.

> A lot of people think peanuts or almond butter are great protein sources, and start their day with them. But here's the truth: they do have protein, but they have way more fat than protein! They are actually **50–55 per cent fat and only ~20–25 per cent protein.**
>
> Peanuts and dry fruits are fine as snacks, but don't rely on them as your primary protein source. Since they're higher in fat, eating too much can lead to weight gain. Balance is key!

'If protein is so essential, can I just eat protein-rich foods? Will all my problems go away? Will I build muscle?'

This is an incredibly common and valid question, especially in an era dominated by fitness trends and quick-fix diets. The simple answer is no, not entirely. While protein is undeniably a powerhouse macronutrient, it cannot solve every dietary problem on its own, and an excessive focus on it can even be detrimental.

To understand how to use protein effectively, we need to identify the sources of protein and consider three key aspects: *how much* to eat, *when* to eat it, and *how* to include it in a healthy diet.

Protein's role in muscle building is clear, but that process requires more than just high intake. It necessitates a synergy with carbohydrates for energy and recovery, healthy fats for hormone regulation, and a variety of vitamins and minerals to facilitate all the underlying metabolic processes. Relying solely on protein-rich foods risks creating nutritional deficiencies and placing undue stress on the kidneys. Therefore, before attempting to overhaul your diet with a protein-only focus, let's explore the fundamental building blocks of this essential nutrient and establish the necessary context for its proper consumption.

Protein needs to work with carbs for energy and recovery, with healthy fats for hormones, and with vitamins and minerals for body processes. Eating only protein can lead one to miss out on other nutrients and can impair one's digestion and gut health. So, before changing your diet to make it all about protein, we'll look at what protein is and how to eat it correctly.

Vegetarian Foods	**Protein/100 grams**
Soyabean, White	37.8
Pulses (Masoor, Moong, Chana, etc.)	22–25
Rajma	19.5
Chana	21.1
Black-Eyed Peas	21
Paneer	18.8
Tofu	15.8
Sprouted Legumes	8–10
Curd	10

Table 1.2: *Protein content in vegetarian foods*

Non-Vegetarian Foods	Protein/100 grams
Chicken	31
Fish	18–22
Eggs	6–12
Prawns	19
Goat Meat/Mutton	20–21

Table 1.3: *Protein content in non-vegetarian foods*

Now, let's discuss our daily protein requirement. Using the example diet (Table 1.1), consisting of roti, vegetables and dal-rice, we will explore ways to increase protein intake by adding protein-rich ingredients. It is important to remember that most people who are not professional athletes do not need to meticulously weigh their food. Measuring by volume is a good, practical alternative and a significant improvement over simply eating a 'roti-sabzi' lunch.

Let's see how much protein can be included in a regular diet if we pay some attention to protein content when choosing our food.

If we add an egg to the popular breakfast of tea and poha, we can easily boost the protein content by 6 grams. Likewise, pairing a fistful of peanuts with vada pav gives us an additional 7 grams of protein. This doesn't imply that vada pav is a healthy choice, but I will humour vada pav lovers for the time being. For dinner, if we include some paneer or just plain chicken with dal and rice, there's no need for a curry or gravy; even grilled chicken can add around 20–21 grams of protein. Do note that I'm not suggesting this as a perfect healthy diet. This is simply to illustrate the concept of protein-forward thinking.

Food Item	Protein (in Grams)	Other Protein Sources	Quantity	Protein (in Grams)	Total Protein (in Grams)
Poha + Tea (Breakfast)	4.5	Egg	1	6	10.5
Vegetable + Wheat Roti (Lunch)	3	Lentils	1.5 bowls	6	9
Tea + Vada Pav	1.5	Peanuts	1 fistful	7	8.5
Rice + Lentils (thin dal) (Dinner)	3	Paneer/ Chicken	1.5 bowls/100 grams	21	24
Total Protein	**12**			**40**	**52**

Table 1.4: *Protein intake through the day*

What Does Protein-Forward Thinking Mean?

To support your health, it's important to aim for at least 0.8–1 gram of protein for every kilogram of body weight. While 55–60 grams of protein might seem like a small amount, reaching that goal daily can be tough. Do remember that there is a very common misconception that 100 grams of chicken or paneer gives you 100 grams of protein. We have already seen in the previous tables that it is not so. How, then, to eat the optimal quantity of protein? In each meal—whether you have 3 or 4 meals a day—try to include at least 10 grams of protein. I know, I know! You are going to come at me with 'What? Just 10 grams of protein in every meal? That's only 40 grams of protein!' Yes, I know. But hear me out. You saw the dismal protein levels that most people's diets are at, right? I also showed you how protein-deficient our entire population is? So, we agree that it is a problem to be tackled. But when it comes to problems or challenges, we know from experience that be it savings or SIP, or protein in meals, it is always best to start small. When you keep your starting goal a little small, it is easier to consistently achieve it every day. Once the baseline has moved up, and in this case, the daily protein intake has moved up from 10 grams per day to 40 grams per day, we can easily take it to 60, 70 or 80 grams of protein per day, as by then, our body and mind will be used to thinking about and eating protein-rich food regularly, at every meal.

Coming back to our 1 gram of protein per kilogram of body weight, sure, 55–60 grams of protein a day sounds easy, but what happens when you actually try to hit that target daily? You will quickly realise that it is not as easy as it seems.

So, where do you start?

Whatever you're eating (whether it's three or four meals a day), ensure each meal provides at least 10 grams of protein. For example, you could include:

- A small chicken breast
- About a cup of cooked rajma
- 1.5 cups of dahi
- Half a cup of paneer bhurji

Now, if you do the math, if you're only getting 10 grams per meal and eating three times a day, you're still falling short, hitting only 30 grams of protein. But remember what I told you: start small. One step at a time is a better way to succeed than a giant leap. And just upping your protein game a little like this can make a huge difference in your health.

Once you have achieved the basics of consuming 10 grams of protein in each meal, give yourself the task of increasing it to 15 grams per meal, and eventually you will find that eating an adequate amount of protein, planning for it, thinking about whether you are getting any protein from the food in front of you, and so on, is, what I call, **'protein-forward thinking'**!

The best part? Even if I end up having just aloo parathas for breakfast—which, for the record, barely have any protein—I'll still keep in mind that I need to compensate for that protein shortfall at lunch.

Change your mindset, and your eating habits will naturally follow. That's the key to building lasting habits! So, the next time you're planning your meal, don't start with carbs. Instead, begin with what protein to include and then figure out the rest.

Now let's explore what a protein-forward diet looks like. And no, vada pav isn't on the list now!

Vegetarian Diet

Meal	Menu	Quantity (grams)	Proteins (grams)
Breakfast	1 fistful of walnuts		4
	1 cup milk	250	8
	2 moong dal chilla (made from 50 grams soaked moong dal)	200	10
	1 banana	50	0.6
Lunch	1 wholewheat phulka	30	3.3
	100 grams paneer sabzi	104	18
	1 cup french beans sabzi	100	2
	1 cup raita made with curd	150	3
Evening snacks	0.5 cup boiled chana chaat	15	3.5
Dinner	1 cup masoor pulao	30	8
	salad	50	1
	1 glass buttermilk	200	3
Total			**69.4 grams**

Table 1.5: *Vegetarian diet for a day*

For breakfast, if you include foods like walnuts, milk and moong dal chilla, you'll get around 4 grams of protein from walnuts, 8 grams from milk, and 10 grams from the moong dal chilla.

For lunch and dinner, pairing wholewheat phulkas with a protein-rich paneer curry or other protein sources like chickpeas, sprouted lentils, kidney beans or soybeans will help you meet your daily protein needs.

'But Amita, how can we eat dal or legumes every single day?' This is a common question. My answer to that is: 'The same way you're always ready to eat potatoes every day. No complaints there, right?'

Vegetarian Diet and Protein

Many vegetarian people come to me asking for ways to stop hair fall and boost energy, and they also want to avoid protein powders. Yet these same vegetarian individuals refuse to eat dal, legumes, paneer or soya regularly. How can this work? Vegetarian diets can already be challenging for meeting one's daily protein needs, and protein is the very foundation of all our tissues and energy cycles. If you consistently skip key vegetarian protein sources like pulses, beans, lentils and dairy, improving your health becomes practically impossible.

> Soybeans are an excellent protein source—especially for vegetarians!
>
> Soybeans contain 52 grams of protein per 100 grams. Soybeans also have a unique distinction of being a plant-based food with all the essential amino acids.
>
> Before you start counting a small bowl of soybeans curry as protein-rich, here's something to remember:
>
> When soaked and cooked with veggies, 30 grams of soybeans expands to about one and a half cups. That means in just one meal, you're getting around 16 grams of protein from soybeans alone. This is fantastic, but remember the amount that you need to eat. Taking half a small bowl of soybean curry and assuming that you are getting 16 grams of protein is incorrect.
>
> Is it okay to eat soybeans with hypothyroidism? Yes! You can include soybeans two to three times a week in your diet. They're actually beneficial for hormonal health and are packed with fibre too![10]

> **Curd vs. buttermilk**
>
> Curd is a source of lactose, a type of carbohydrate, and it contains around 10 grams of protein per 100 grams. However, it's not a rich protein source like paneer or chicken, so don't expect it to do the heavy lifting for your protein needs.
>
> That said, every bit of protein counts, so take it where you can! Plus, yogurt also provides B12 and D3, two essential nutrients primarily found in animal-based foods.
>
> When you make buttermilk from yogurt, its nutrients don't disappear! However, if you dilute 100 grams of yogurt too much, and drink just one glass, you're getting fewer probiotics and less protein.
>
> For a good probiotic boost, aim for at least two glasses of buttermilk. That way, you're actually reaping the benefits.
>
> Buttermilk or yogurt does NOT cause joint pain. Some people have a sensitivity to sour foods, which *might* cause discomfort, but that's not the case for everyone. In fact, many people who blame yogurt for their knee pain are often protein deficient!
>
> Pro Tip: These days, you'll find high-protein curd or yogurt in the market. If you have no issues digesting dairy, you can easily include it in your daily diet. Most of these yogurts contain around 12 grams of protein per 100 grams, making them a solid option for boosting your protein intake!

Non-Vegetarian Diet and Protein

If you are a vegetarian, do not skip reading this part. As you will realise, even for those who eat non-vegetarian food, if they don't plan their meals carefully, they will struggle as much as vegetarians to meet their protein requirements.

A fun fact about Indian non-vegetarians: they are barely eating enough meat or chicken to actually get enough protein. Most non-vegetarian families of four end up cooking only 500 grams of chicken or mutton on the bone. That leaves them with barely 50 grams of actual meat or chicken per person, that too provided it is equally divided between everyone. The majority of women or young girls will often end up eating mostly curry and very little of the actual meat. This explains why most of us continue to be protein-deficient even when we apparently have a large meat-eating population in our country.[11]

Let's take a real look at how much chicken or fish one actually needs. And no, I'm not talking about that oily chicken curry with a spoonful of gravy; I am talking about the actual chicken pieces!

Meal	**Menu**	**Quantity (Grams)**	**Protein (Grams)**
Breakfast	1 Egg Omelette	50	6.5
	2 Wholewheat Phulkas	60	6.6
Lunch	1 Cup Cooked Rice	30	3.1
	100 grams Fish Curry	100	21.5
	1 Cup Salad	100	2
Evening Snacks	1 Fruit, Orange	100	-
	1 Fistful of Almonds + Walnuts	7.5	3
Dinner	2 Wholewheat Phulkas	60	6.6
	1 Cup Chole Curry	30	7
	1 Cup Ladies Finger Sabzi	100	2
	1 Cup Salad	50	1
Total			**60 grams**

Table 1.6: *Non-vegetarian diet for a day.*

For breakfast, an egg omelette with wholewheat rotis is a fantastic option, packing in 13.1 grams of protein. If you're vegetarian on a particular day, swap the eggs for paneer paratha or moong dal chilla—still a solid protein start!

For lunch, a fish curry with rice can give you around 24.6 grams of protein. On a meatless day, you can opt for rajma-rice or soybean sabzi with wholewheat roti, which are great vegetarian alternatives.

For an evening snack, pairing an orange with almonds and walnuts gives you 7.5 grams of protein. Not into nuts? No problem! Swap them for makhana (fox nuts) or boiled chickpeas.

For dinner, a meal of wholewheat rotis, masoor dal and bhindi sabzi provides 15.6 grams of protein. Want an even better protein boost? Add a yogurt-based raita or go for a moong dal khichdi—comfort food that works!

Can we eat eggs daily?

You can safely eat two whole eggs every day—no need to ditch the yolk! And eating two eggs a day DOES NOT make your entire diet high in protein! All generally healthy people can eat two whole eggs per day. There's no need to separate the yellow from your eggs. The concern about the cholesterol in egg yolk increasing your blood cholesterol levels is also misplaced. Eating cholesterol doesn't spike your blood cholesterol. It's your total fat intake that plays a bigger role in raising cholesterol levels![12]

For bodybuilders who need extra protein, add six to ten extra egg whites to their diet.

Does protein rich food lose its protein content on cooking?

When you cook protein-rich foods like eggs, their protein structure changes. This process is called denaturation. But don't worry, this doesn't destroy the protein!

You don't need to eat raw eggs to get the benefits. In fact, cooked eggs are easier to digest because the protein becomes solid and more bioavailable for your body. So, go ahead—scramble, boil or eat a sunny side up!

Does cheese give us protein?

Yes, cheese *does* contain protein, but it's not exactly a *high-protein* food. Why? Because it also comes loaded with fat and sodium.

Take Parmesan, for example. 100 grams has about 38 grams of protein, sure, but also 29 grams of fat. Even low-fat paneer gives you 20 grams of protein with around 22 grams of fat.

And don't even get me started on processed cheese. Many of them contain hydrogenated vegetable oils as emulsifiers, which sneak in trans fats. What are trans fats? We'll get to that in the next chapter.

But for now, just know this—that layer of gooey processed cheese being dumped over *everything* these days is not doing your health any favour. And if you're eating it thinking it's your protein source, then don't be surprised if your next stop is the cardiologist's clinic. And, *no*, your cheese dosa does not count as a high-protein food!

So, does that mean you should *never* eat cheese? No, that's not what I'm saying. But what kind of cheese you're eating matters.

For example, feta cheese is lower in fat and, texture-wise, quite similar to paneer. It can be a better choice, especially if eaten in moderation and combined with whole grains or veggies.

But remember, cheese alone can't meet your daily protein needs. You'll still need your dals, eggs, tofu, fish or chicken to hit your protein goals for the day.

Tips to maximise dietary proteins

1. Choose high-protein foods such as chicken, seafood, paneer, eggs, tofu, soybeans, lentils and legumes.
2. Ensure that every meal includes a source of protein.
3. Meal planning helps in stocking up on protein sources in advance or soaking them beforehand. Preparing ahead ensures that you get enough protein in every meal.
4. If you have a busy schedule and cannot plan each meal, consider taking protein supplements. Just make sure they do not contain heavy metals beyond permissible limits, excessive food additives, caffeine, sugar, excessive multivitamins, minerals or artificial flavours.

How Will I Know if I Am Getting Enough Protein?

'Amita, just like we test for B12 or D3 levels, can we test for protein levels in the blood? Can a blood test tell us if we're getting enough protein from our diet?'

I love this question because it comes from a very scientific perspective! Here's the thing: there's no direct test to check if you're eating enough protein. And that's because when you don't get enough protein from food, your body simply dips into its own protein reserves. And what are those reserves? Your muscles!

So even if you're not consuming enough protein, your body keeps running by breaking down muscle tissue. That means your body might be silently struggling long before any blood test picks it up.

However, once the 'protein drought' starts taking a toll on your health, we can detect it through indirect tests like Total Protein, Serum Albumin, Prealbumin (Transthyretin), and Albumin-Globulin Ratio.[13] But by the time these tests show any abnormalities, the damage is already done! So, think of it like checking how bad a drought has got rather than predicting when it will hit.

The best way to track whether you're getting enough protein? Keep a **food diary**! Write down your protein sources and use a food-tracking app to keep tabs on your intake. Simple, effective and way more reliable than waiting for a blood test to sound the alarm!

Another way to spot a protein deficiency? Look for the signs and symptoms.

If you're feeling tired all the time, your wounds take forever to heal, your muscles feel weak, your nails are brittle, your hair is falling out, you can't focus, your immunity is low, or you're dealing with constant mood swings—your body might be screaming for more protein!

Also, if you're experiencing these symptoms, you should consult a doctor or a nutritionist and increase your protein intake. But remember to get it checked out as these signs aren't exclusive to protein deficiency. Conditions like anemia can show similar symptoms.

That said, in most people, if there's a micronutrient deficiency, there's a high chance they're also lacking protein. So don't ignore the signs.

Do You Need More Protein if You Work Out Regularly?

Your protein needs depend on your weight, goals and workout intensity. If you're lifting heavy weights, your protein requirement goes up to support muscle repair and growth.

Bodybuilders aim for hypertrophy (muscle gain), which is why they consume a lot of eggs and high-protein foods, especially non-vegetarian sources, which are naturally protein-rich and have a complete amino acid profile.

But if you're just doing basic workouts at the gym, you don't need to overload on eggs or chicken. A balanced diet with moderate protein intake is enough to support your fitness goals!

Protein Supplements: What's the Deal?

The word 'supplement' means something that is extra and not the main deal. In the context of nutrition, supplement means something that is not our primary food, not the regular diet we consume, but something that can further support us in case of a gap. A protein supplement is one such example.

Does everyone need a protein supplement? Nope! If your diet is on point and you're getting all the protein you need from food, you're good to go, no supplement required.

But let's be real, if you barely eat, don't have time to cook, can't stomach large meals, or are always on the move with no access to protein-rich food, then, yes, a supplement makes sense.

Or if your workout routine has increased, why do trainers often recommend protein? Because most people's diets are protein-deficient.

Why do we go to the gym? To build muscle! Whether you want to grow muscle or make your existing muscles stronger, you need protein. Muscles are made of protein; they can't be built from fat, carbs or glucose.

Can't We Get Enough Protein from Our Daily Meals? Why Is a Supplement Necessary?

Of course, we can meet all our protein requirements from food, but if you are unable to eat properly due to some reasons like travel, a busy schedule, lack of availability of protein-rich foods, or any other reasons, there is absolutely no harm in, nor should there be any guilt about, opting for a protein supplement.

Now, if you need to consume 70 grams of protein in a day, you'd have to eat at least 300–400 grams of chicken. Many people mistakenly believe that eating 100 grams of chicken gives them 100 grams of protein, but that's not true.

Remember 100 grams of chicken only provides around 24–25 grams of protein.

Other foods like yogurt also contain protein but how much yogurt do we actually eat? A spoonful? Two? Maybe half a cup? If you want to rely on yogurt as a primary protein source, you'd need to eat at least 200 grams of high-protein yogurt. Regular yogurt doesn't have a lot of protein. The high-protein variants available in the market today usually provide around 16 grams of protein per 200-gram pack.

So, the point is, you can get enough protein from food, but only if you track it carefully and plan your diet well. If you're working out but not giving your body the fuel it needs, you'll struggle. You might feel weak, see no progress, lift the same weights for months, and wonder why your strength isn't improving. The simple reason? You're not getting enough protein!

The most important thing—you can track how much protein you're consuming! Nowadays, there are many apps available for this. Simply enter the foods you eat (like two eggs for breakfast or a bowl of dal for lunch), and the app will estimate your total daily protein intake. Even ChatGPT does a decent job!

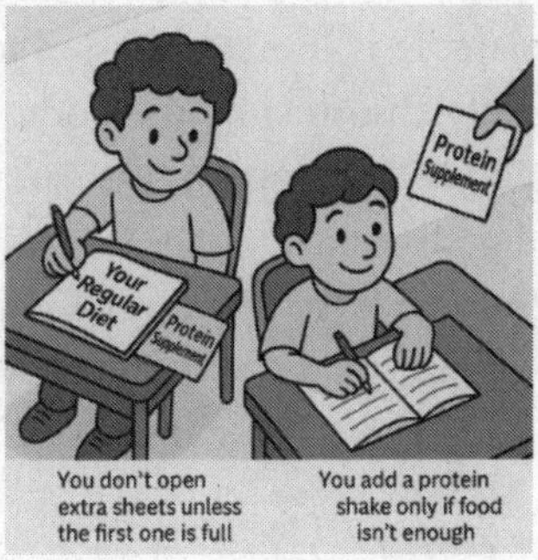
Protein Supplement
Your Regular Diet
Protein Supplement
You don't open extra sheets unless the first one is full
You add a protein shake only if food isn't enough

Image 1.2: *The 'Extra Sheet' rule for protein*

A protein supplement is just that—a supplement. Think of it like extra answer sheets during an exam; you only take them when your main answer book is full. Similarly, you should only consider a protein supplement if your diet isn't providing enough protein. If you start having protein shakes twice a day without any real need, two things can happen—your body could get digestive stress, and you might miss out on other essential nutrients. This can even lead to constipation!

There are two types of protein supplements: whey protein and plant-based protein.

Whey protein is derived from milk. It's the leftover liquid when paneer is made from milk. This liquid is then processed by removing water, concentrating the protein, and converting it into powder.

Plant-based protein comes from sources like rice, soybeans, peas and quinoa. The carbohydrates are removed from these sources to make the protein easier to digest.

1. Whey Protein: This is derived from milk.
    a. Whey Concentrate: It contains lactose, so it is not suitable for those with lactose intolerance.
    b. Whey Isolate: It is more processed and lactose-free, and is quickly absorbed by the body.
    c. Whey Hydrolyzed Protein: It is easier to digest as it contains digestive enzymes.
    d. Casein Protein: It is the slowest-digesting protein, and is beneficial for muscle recovery when taken at night.

Pro Tip: Instead of discarding the leftover water while making paneer, use it for kneading dough; it's a natural source of whey protein, albeit a very diluted one!

Plant protein comes from sources like peanuts, soy, peas, quinoa, moong and hemp.

- The most popular plant-based options in the market are soy protein and pea protein. Select one based on your taste and budget.
- If you experience digestive issues or have trouble with lactose, plant protein is an excellent alternative!

Protein supplements aren't a miracle solution; they play a supportive role in your overall diet. The key is to obtain natural protein from a well-rounded diet. Prioritise whole foods, and consider supplements only as a secondary option when necessary!

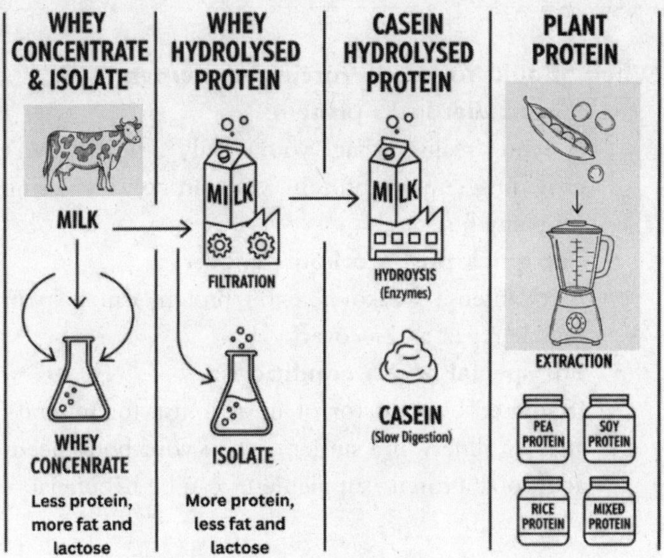

Image 1.3: *Sources of protein supplements*

What is yeast protein?

Yeast protein is a high-quality, plant-based protein derived from nutritional or brewer's yeast (usually Saccharomyces cerevisiae). After yeast cells grow on nutrient-rich media (like molasses), they're harvested, dried and processed. The result is a protein concentrate or isolate that's neutral in taste and free from active yeast, so it doesn't cause fermentation or bloating. It's also easy to digest and naturally contains B vitamins, zinc and immune-supporting beta-glucans.[14] Since it's vegan, dairy-free, gluten-free and soy-free, it suits almost everyone. With a mild taste, it can easily be added to smoothies, soups, parathas or pancakes to boost their protein content without changing their flavour. In short, it gives you the power of whey, minus the dairy.

When Should You Use Protein Supplements?

- **If your diet lacks protein:**
  If you realise that your daily meals aren't providing enough protein, you can consider using supplements.
- **For quick post-workout recovery:**
  After intense workouts, extra protein can help in muscle repair and recovery.
- **For special health conditions:**
  If advised by a doctor or nutritionist, for instance, after an illness or a surgery when your body needs additional protein, supplements can be beneficial.

Do Children Need to Take Protein Powders for Better Growth?

I don't recommend protein supplements for children unless they are clinically undernourished, and are not gaining weight or are unable to eat. As a general rule, children need to be meeting their protein requirements from only the food they eat. You don't even need to be giving things like protein bars to young children as their protein requirements are really very low. The real protein deficiency in the urban population begins at adolescence. Although even for adolescent children, the focus should be on ensuring variety in their diet and not supplementation.

Do I Only Need to Take a Protein Supplement if I Am Going to the Gym?

We adults—women and men—become too busy with the demands of our busy lives and neglect our diet. This, in turn, leads to all the health problems that protein deficiency brings along with it.

When people begin their gym journey, they quickly notice the increased energy demands of their bodies due to a boost in strength. A balanced diet can enhance workout performance, and exercise raises the body's need for protein. This is why people opt for protein supplements once they start working out.

However, most protein supplements in the market are not ideal for children, women or the elderly. For instance, many children's and women's protein powders can contain as much as 70 per cent sugar, which is not desirable. Thus, it is crucial to verify the actual protein content and check the additives in these supplements. Likewise, women's protein powders often have unnecessary additives, such as herbal ingredients, high sugar levels, or maltodextrin.

What to Consider When Buying a Protein Supplement

Before you buy protein powder, always take a look at the ingredients!

- First, it should be free of added sugars.
- Second, opt for a protein concentrate or a mix of concentrate and isolate.
- Sweeteners like stevia or erythritol are acceptable, but steer clear of too many anti-caking agents.
- Pick a reputable brand that features a hologram and has positive reviews.
- Also, keep in mind who is recommending the protein to you!

Many gym trainers promote protein powders, but some may include harmful ingredients or lack the required quality. Make sure it doesn't contain heavy metals like arsenic or lead, as these can pose health risks.

How to Choose a Protein Supplement?

First, determine why you need a protein supplement. Is it for muscle building, overall health, or muscle recovery?

Based on your preferences and budget, choose from whey, casein, isolate or plant-based protein.

If you have allergies or food intolerances, consider choosing plant-based protein instead of whey or whey isolate.

Make sure you carefully examine the nutrition label. Look for any excessive food additives, caffeine, sugar or high amounts of multivitamins. Additionally, verify that it offers a sufficient amount of protein per gram.

Some individuals may find protein powder difficult to digest. If that's the case, you might want to try hydrolyzed protein or protein isolates.

If you can fulfil your daily protein requirements through whole foods, there's no need for protein supplements. Keep in mind that protein supplements are primarily for convenience—they can help bridge gaps in your dietary protein intake, but they shouldn't replace meals.

Can People with Diabetes Take Protein Supplements?

In diabetes management, it's not just about controlling carbohydrate intake; maintaining a balance of protein and fibre is equally important.

Including protein in meals can help reduce the spike in glucose levels after eating. So, try to slightly reduce carbohydrate intake and add good protein sources and fibre to your meals. Normally, glucose levels rise after meals, but consuming protein and fibre-rich foods helps slow down this spike, leading to better blood sugar control.

Even if you have diabetes, you can take protein supplements. However, the right amount depends on your total calorie intake and weight.

Does Eating More Protein Increase Uric Acid?

Uric acid levels do not increase due to protein, but rather because of foods high in purines. Protein and purines are as different as chalk and cheese.

Foods high in purines include alcohol (especially beer) and seafood like lobster, crab and prawns. Additionally, consuming too much fruit juice, tonics or beverages with high-fructose corn syrup can also raise uric acid levels.

If you have type 2 diabetes (T2DM), high BP, or have been overweight for a long time, your risk of gout and high uric acid levels increases. Dehydration can also contribute to elevated uric acid.

So, instead of blaming protein, focus on reducing purine-rich foods.

If your uric acid levels are high, cutting down on protein completely may actually slow down your healing process.

Do Protein Supplements Put Stress on the Kidneys?

As mentioned earlier, if protein powder (whey or plant protein) comes from natural food sources, how could it lead to kidney stones? Just take a look at the ingredients and steer clear of those with excessive food additives or caffeine. However, if you have existing kidney problems or a history of kidney stones, it's important to monitor your total protein intake. If you take five scoops of protein each day, do no drink enough water, neglect exercise, and do not maintain a balanced diet, and if you continue doing this for an extended period of time, it could affect your kidneys.[15] But the standard recommendation for a protein supplement is one to two scoops per day. Beyond that, for most non-athlete adults, it is recommended that they focus on getting the remaining protein from food.

Do You Need to Take Protein Powder Immediately After Exercise?

Many people believe that optimising the 'recovery window' is crucial for muscle recovery and synthesis.

A comprehensive study showed that while there might be a slight benefit to muscle growth, further analysis found no significant difference.[16]

The key takeaway is that your total protein intake throughout the day matters more than just increasing protein consumption immediately after a workout.

Can plant protein or (unflavoured) whey isolate be added to paratha dough?

Both plant protein and whey isolate are heat-stable enough for light cooking. When mixed into paratha dough, they boost the protein content of your meal without altering the taste much (if unflavoured).

Pro Tip: Add 1 tablespoon of protein powder per paratha. You may need to add a little more water while kneading the dough.

Drinking Enough Water Is Important on a High-Protein Diet

- **Supports kidney function:** A high-protein diet increases the workload on the kidneys as they need to remove toxins like urea.[17] Staying hydrated helps them function properly.
- **Aids Digestion:** If you consume more than 25 grams of protein at a time, your body may take longer to digest it. Increasing protein intake gradually, along with sufficient water, helps your digestion adapt.
- **Essential for muscle maintenance:** Proper hydration prevents muscle cramps and fatigue and supports optimal muscle protein synthesis during recovery and growth.

Pro Tip: As you increase protein intake, increase your water intake too!

Do Protein Supplements Cause Bloating, Constipation or Acne?

Many people believe that protein supplements lead to bloating, swelling, constipation or acne, but here's why these issues may occur:

- **Feeling full or bloated**: Protein takes longer to digest than carbs like rice or poha, which can make you feel full for a long time. If protein intake is not balanced with fibre-rich foods like vegetables and lentils, digestion issues may arise.
- **Constipation issues**: Some people consume too much protein but not enough fibre, leading to digestive imbalances. Ensure your diet includes veggies, pulses and enough water to support digestion.
- **Acne and skin issues**: Protein itself does not directly cause acne, but high-fat diets and digestive imbalances can contribute to it. If you have lactose intolerance, consuming whey concentrate (which contains lactose) may lead to bloating, skin breakouts and other gut issues. Switching to plant-based protein or whey isolate (which has less lactose) can help.

Pro Tip: Balance your protein intake with fibre, water and healthy fats to avoid these side effects!

Creatine: The hot new supplement on the block

Creatine is one of the most well-researched and effective supplements. It helps with strength, recovery and performance. It is also useful for menopausal women in that it helps improve their energy, reduces brain fog, and helps to maintain muscle.[18]

But before you even think about it, fix your basics. If your protein and fibre intake is low, start there. Most people don't eat enough of either.

Taking creatine without eating enough protein or fibre is like adding a turbocharger to a car that has no fuel. It looks impressive, but it won't get you very far.

Once your diet is in place, creatine can be a great add-on. It helps your muscles recover faster during short bursts of activity like weight training or sprinting. The best form is creatine monohydrate. A standard dose is around 3 to 5 grams per day, ideally with professional guidance.[19]

As for a few common myths:

- It's not a steroid.
- It doesn't harm healthy kidneys,
- There's no solid evidence linking it to hair loss.[20]

But creatine is only helpful if you are also strength training alongside having a good diet.[21, 22]

Is There Any Relationship Between Hair Fall and Protein?

The most crucial nutrient for hair health is protein. Hair is mainly composed of a protein known as keratin. If your body lacks enough protein (the essential building block), how can it generate new hair?

If you're experiencing hair loss or want to improve hair growth, the first step is to evaluate the protein content in your diet. You don't have to rely on protein supplements; just make sure that each of your three daily meals contains a good source of protein. Just as you need bricks to build a wall, without a source of protein, hair growth becomes challenging.

Nourishing your hair from the inside is crucial. Rather than solely using an egg-based hair mask, consuming eggs is far more advantageous as they supply the body with vital protein and other nutrients, which can help minimise hair loss and promote hair growth.

Your diet should consist of:

- Non-vegetarian options like eggs and chicken
- Dairy and plant-based proteins such as yogurt, paneer, tofu and lentils
- A variety of vegetables
- Healthy fats like almonds, peanuts, coconut and seeds (like sesame and flaxseeds)
- Traditional foods like flaxseeds chutney and whole grains

Now that we have understood that the first pillar of our health and diet is **protein**, let's move on to another nutrient that you have already seen me mention a few times in the book so far: **fibre.**

2

Fibre

Back in 2001, when I first became a student of nutrition, dietary fibre was taught or mentioned as an afterthought. We had general guidelines about fibre and how much of it one 'could' be having each day, but its role or what was taught to us thereof was limited to 'forming bulk for stool'. When I began working with patients in hospitals and community centres, I realised that dietary fibre is probably more important than carbohydrates even! Here's a fact: 70 per cent people in the world or India are eating a diet deficient in fibre.[1,2,3] This has implications ranging from poor immunity to colon cancer!

I truly believe that fibre deserves to be recognised as a macronutrient because adequate fibre intake can help prevent numerous health issues. It is vital for weight loss, weight management, cholesterol control, hormone balance, diabetes, menopause management and immunity. Fibre has a role to play everywhere![4]

In fact, it wouldn't be an overstatement to say that fibre is just as crucial as protein!

What Is Fibre?

Dietary fibre is a type of carbohydrate that our body cannot digest, but it acts as food for some other 'beings' in our body.

It is not absorbed in the small intestine, but it does help the digestive system in functioning properly.

Fibre plays a crucial role in removing waste from the body and maintaining regular bowel movements. That's why, when you experience constipation, foods like guava, cucumber and banana are recommended. They literally get you going!

We get fibre from all the plant-based food that we eat. And no, you do not get any fibre from tough, fibrous-looking chicken. This was an actual misunderstanding of a patient of mine, I swear I am not making it up!

Fibre is mainly of two types:

- **Soluble fibre:** This dissolves in water to form a gel-like substance. It helps lower cholesterol, regulates blood sugar levels, and improves heart health. Some types of soluble fibre like fructans (found in vegetables and root vegetables) and galactans (found in fruits) also act as 'food' for the bacteria in our gut, called gut microbiome. More on this later.
- **Insoluble fibre:** This does not dissolve in water and adds bulk to the stool, helping prevent constipation, improve digestion, and prevent colon cancer.

Both kinds of fibre are equally important for our body and gut health. So, it helps to generally eat more fibre in the form of plant-based food, rather than obsess over the type of fibre one is eating. Thankfully, nature does not discriminate, and we find fibre in *all* plant-based foods without an exception.

How Does Fibre Actually Work?

We have understood what fibre is, but how does it really work? To understand that, we are going to have to use our imagination. Let's imagine that fibre (soluble and insoluble alike) and other nutrients (protein, carbohydrates, fats, vitamins and minerals) are all playing a game of 'human train' or 'train under a tunnel' like little children do.

If one kid suddenly starts running too fast or in the wrong direction, the others quickly bring them back in line. If another kid gets too disruptive or spoils the game for others, they're pushed out of the game altogether.

Fibre works a bit like that, helping regulate and balance how nutrients move and behave in your digestive system. It slows down things that are going too fast (like sugar absorption), helps eliminate what's unnecessary or harmful, and keeps the whole digestive 'game' smooth and in order.

1. When the carbohydrates in our food start raising blood sugar levels too quickly, soluble fibre steps in to slow things down.[5] Think of it like this, soluble fibre forms a gel. This gel traps sugar and starch molecules inside it. This slows down their absorption, so the sugar enters the bloodstream gradually, in what we call a *sustained release* manner. Because the sugar isn't flooding the bloodstream all at once, blood glucose levels stay more stable. And when your glucose control is good, your HbA1c levels (your average blood sugar over three months) also stay in check. Now if you're trying to manage diabetes, this stability is exactly what you need. That's why fibre plays such an important role. In fact, this is why we always ask people with diabetes to *add vegetables to every meal*, or to *mix other pulses or millets along*

with rice or wheat. For example, add soybean or flaxseed to your roti dough, make parathas stuffed with veggies, or add lots of vegetables to your khichdi. These little tweaks can go a long way in managing your blood sugar better, all thanks to fibre.

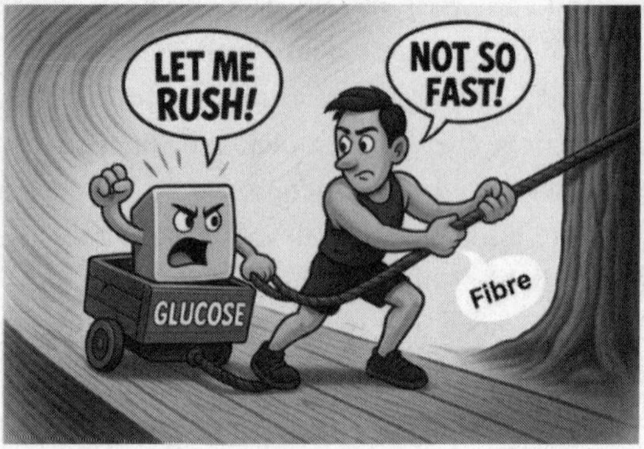

Image 2.1: *Fibre slowing down sugar consumption*

Remember Kids Playing 'Human Train'? That's Food in the Gut!

Everything we eat first enters the stomach, mixes with acids and enzymes, and forms a soft, mushy paste. This paste, called chyme, is then slowly pushed forward towards the small intestine.

This forward movement of food is called **peristalsis**—somewhat like the 'train' we talked about. The food needs to keep moving along smoothly. If it stalls in one place for too long—which is what happens when you have been 'backed up' for a few days—the cells lining the gut can get irritated or even damaged. And if that keeps happening day after day, year after year, your risk of developing **colon cancer** goes up. In fact, people who eat less than 10 grams of fibre a day have *up to an 18 per cent* higher risk of colon cancer.[6] Why? Because fibre adds **bulk** to your food, and that bulk keeps the digestive train moving. Without enough fibre, your digestion is like driving a car with constant braking. And just like constant braking ruins your ride experience, low fibre ruins your gut health experience.

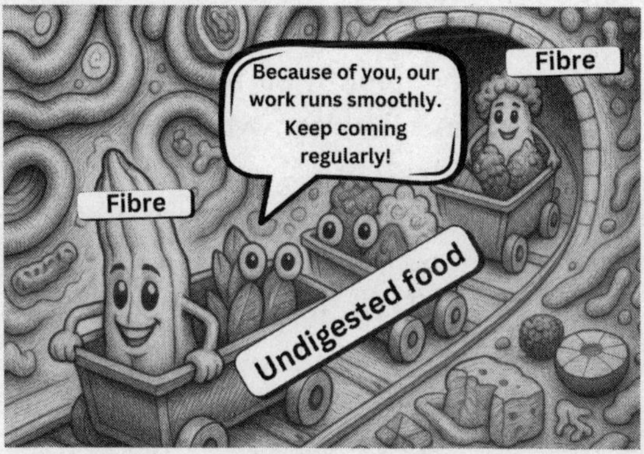
Because of you, our work runs smoothly. Keep coming regularly!
Fibre
Fibre
Undigested food

Image 2.2: *Fibre: the engine of digestion*

Fibre's Most Important Job? Keeping Things *Moving*

Fibre plays a key role in helping food move smoothly through our digestive system—that's actually its most important function.

Remember our 'human train' example with kids? If one kid suddenly stops in the middle, the others behind them give a little push to keep the game going. Fibre does exactly that: it keeps the food bulk moving forward. The time it takes for food to travel through your entire digestive system is called **gastric transit time**. Now, this transit time shouldn't be too fast, but it also shouldn't be too slow. If it's too quick, nutrients don't get absorbed properly. If it's too slow, it can cause gas, constipation, piles, or even lead to vitamin and mineral deficiencies over time.

So if you want to protect your long-term gut health, **fibre needs to be part of every single meal**, no matter what diet you follow.

In any group of kids playing train, there's always that one kid who doesn't follow the rules and disrupts everyone else, and eventually, they're pushed out of the game. Similarly, in our body, certain substances, when present in excess, can become troublemakers. For example, substances like **cholesterol** and **bile acids**. Fibre, especially soluble fibre, traps these using its gel-like structure and helps remove them from the body. That's why when you increase your fibre intake, it not only improves digestion but also **lowers your risk of heart disease** by helping eliminate these 'naughty elements' before they cause harm.[7]

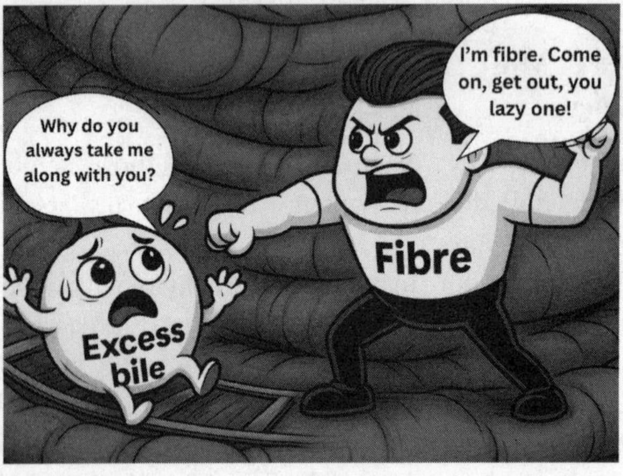
I'm fibre. Come on, get out, you lazy one!
Why do you always take me along with you?
Fibre
Excess bile

Image 2.3: *Fibre helps excrete excess bile*

When too many kids play together, someone has to take the lead. Otherwise, there's chaos. The same goes for your digestion and overall health. And the *unexpected leader* of this whole game? It's something called your **gut microbiome**, the colony of bacteria, yeasts, and other tiny microbes that live in your large intestine, especially in the colon. This microbiome silently oversees many of your body's important functions, from digestion and immunity to mental health. It actually decides *how* things happen and in *which direction* they go. And guess what this leader thrives on? **Soluble fibre.**[8] Fibre is the primary food for your gut microbes, it keeps them happy, diverse and balanced.

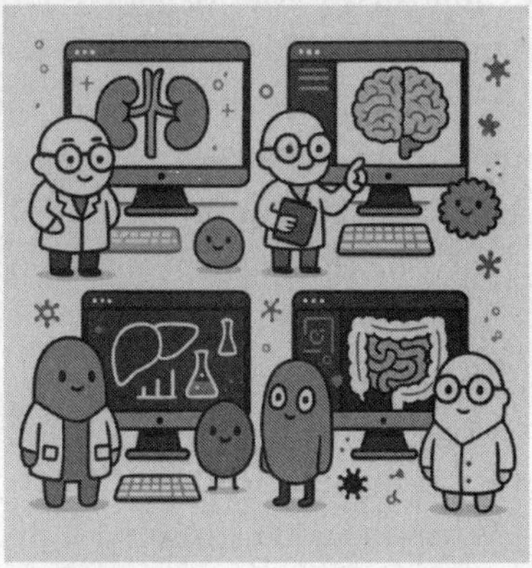

Image 2.4: *Fibre acts like the software running your body's entire operating system*

When you eat enough fibre, the *good bacteria* in your gut, your **gut microbiome**, start to thrive. And when that happens, everything else starts falling into place. Your **mood** improves, your **immunity** gets stronger and even your **hormones** stay more balanced.[9,10,11] If protein is like your **salary**, then fibre is your **health insurance**. You may not notice its effect immediately, but without it, you're constantly at risk. Fibre quietly does the background work to keep your body functioning at its best, and you only realise its value when it's missing.

Why Is Fibre Important?

Including fibre in your daily diet provides several benefits:

- **Improves digestion:**
  Fibre enhances bowel movement, helping relieve constipation.
- **Regulates blood sugar and cholesterol:**
  Soluble fibre helps control blood sugar levels and reduce cholesterol. That's why doctors recommend eating oats for diabetes and heart conditions.
- **Prevents chronic diseases:**
  Regular fibre intake reduces the risk of heart disease, diabetes and cancer. In fact, people who consume less than 10 grams of fibre per day have an 18 per cent higher risk of colon cancer!
- **Improves gut health:**
  We know that the soluble fibre acts as food for the gut bacteria. When the good gut bacteria are kept well fed, they also help our overall health and metabolic balance.
- **Improves mental health:**
  The gut and brain are connected via the enteric nervous system (our gut's very own nervous system), and hence there's a direct feedback loop that our brain and mind work on—a response that originates from the gut. So, if our gut is happy because of the prebiotics in our food, our brain and mind are also going to be happy and calm.[12] Ever experienced

being angry or irritated due to constipation? That happens because the gut is backed up!

- **Improves skin:**
  A large number of skin issues are linked with our gut. When our digestion has gone for a toss, it tends to show on our face and skin. The one guaranteed way of keeping our digestion running smoothly is eating enough fibre.

What Happens if You Don't Get Enough Fibre?

During a clinical internship in Nagpur, also famous for the high concentration of 'piles clinics', I witnessed firsthand the stark consequences of a low-fibre diet. With piles clinics on almost every street, the hot, dry climate, combined with a local diet heavy on spicy curries, sun-dried foods and scant fresh vegetables, created the perfect environment for a surge in conditions like **piles (hemorrhoids)** and **fissures**. Even then, it was clear: a simple increase in dietary **fibre** could have prevented the suffering and the need for surgery in countless patients. Yet the prevailing mindset was 'It's just piles, let's operate', overlooking prevention entirely.

A group of leading Indian gut health experts say constipation is quite common in India. Different community studies show anywhere between 10 and 25 per cent of people may be affected, depending on how constipation is defined and which region is studied. Because many people don't report it, the real number could be even higher.[13] Kolkata is known as India's piles *and* acidity capital. The root cause of this epidemic of constipation, piles and hemorrhoids is the same: a critical **lack of fibre in the diet.** Fibre is not optional; it is the fundamental support structure for a healthy gut. Ignore it, and your body will inevitably show you why it matters.

Problems Caused by a Lack of Fibre in the Diet

1. **Constipation and Digestive Issues:** Constipation is often taken lightly, but chronic constipation significantly increases the risk of colon cancer.[14] Not just that, it can also lead to piles, fissures, hemorrhoids and anal bleeding. The simplest solution to all of these? Increase fibre intake in your diet!
2. **Blood Sugar Instability:** Low fibre intake can cause fluctuations in blood sugar levels, increasing the risk of diabetes.
3. **Increased Risk of Cancer:** A long-term lack of fibre can increase the chances of developing colon cancer.[15]
4. **Weight Gain:** Low fibre consumption leads to overeating, as fibre naturally helps you feel full for longer. Without it, you might end up eating more, leading to weight gain.
5. **Hormonal Imbalance:** Insufficient fibre intake can disrupt hormonal balance, affecting insulin, leptin and other hormones.[16]
6. **Acidity:** Fibre helps remove excess toxins and unwanted substances from the body, including excess stomach acid. A fibre-deficient diet increases acidity, leading to frequent digestive discomfort.

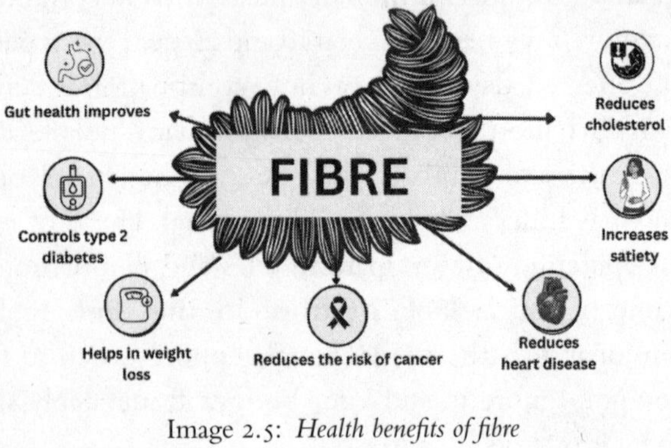

Image 2.5: *Health benefits of fibre*

Where Can You Get Fibre from?

When we talk about fibre, most people immediately think of leafy vegetables or salads. But here's an interesting fact: the highest fibre content is actually found in lentils and legumes![17] Surprised? Well, that's another great reason to include more lentils and legumes in your diet. Do you remember the first benefit of eating lentils? Now you have a second one: dietary fibre!

Sources of Fibre in Our Diet

- Fruits: Apples, oranges, bananas, berries and more
- Vegetables: Broccoli, carrots, cauliflower and beans
- Whole Grains: Jowar (sorghum), bajra (pearl millet) and wholewheat flour
- Legumes: Masoor (red lentils), chickpeas and chana (Bengal gram)
- Nuts and Seeds: Almonds, walnuts, flaxseeds, sesame seeds and others

Isabgol (psyllium husk) is commonly recommended for patients dealing with constipation. It is a well-studied supplement, and taking it daily is generally safe. However, that doesn't mean you can indulge in pizza and biryani at night and expect isabgol to solve all your problems!

If constipation continues even with a balanced diet, taking 1 tablespoon isabgol in two glasses of water after dinner can be a helpful option.[18]

Fibre and Your Gut Health: The Latest Buzzword

Fibre provides nourishment for the beneficial bacteria in your gut, allowing them to flourish.

A healthy gut microbiome—the community of bacteria in your intestines—is essential for a multitude of benefits, including stronger immunity, a balanced mood, increased happiness, improved sleep and proper digestion.

And what do these bacteria love to eat? Fibre!

Fibre provides nourishment, allowing the good bacteria in your gut to flourish. Without sufficient fibre in your diet, taking probiotic foods or supplements is pointless—it's like trying to water an upside-down plant.

What are Probiotics and Prebiotics?

Probiotics: These are beneficial bacteria found in your body, primarily in your gut, that aid in digestion and enhance your immune system. For instance, eating yogurt or buttermilk introduces these helpful bacteria into your body which then form colonies in your gut and help build the microbiome.

Prebiotics: These are types of food, such as fibre, that serve as nourishment for probiotics, allowing them to work more effectively. Foods like bananas, garlic and onions are rich in prebiotics, which promote the growth of good bacteria in your gut.

Think of your digestive system as a garden. The flowers in this garden symbolise the good bacteria (probiotics). To help them thrive, they require fertiliser, which is provided by prebiotics. If you plant flowers (probiotics) and give them the right fertiliser (prebiotics), the garden will flourish beautifully.

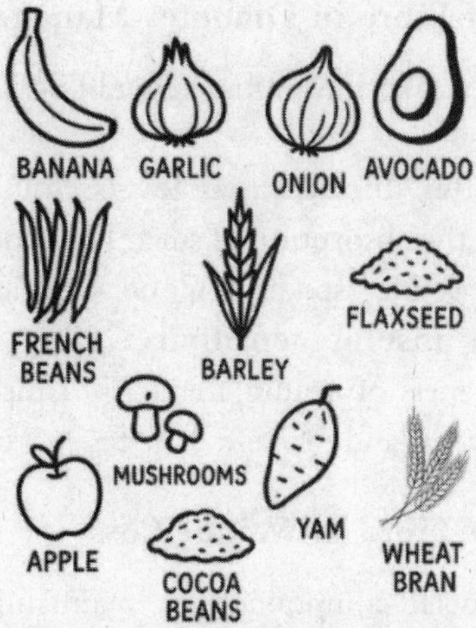

Image 2.6: *Prebiotic Foods Your Body Loves*

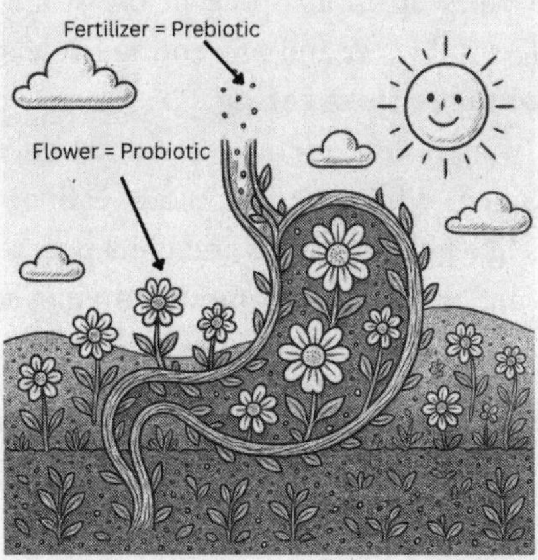

Image 2.7: *The digestive system as a flourishing garden*

In the same way, incorporating probiotic foods like buttermilk and yogurt, along with fibre-rich prebiotics, supports a healthy digestive system!

The Role of Fibre in Diabetes Management

Regular fibre intake aids in managing lifestyle diseases such as diabetes:

- **Regulates blood sugar levels:** Soluble fibre helps to slow the absorption of sugar from food, which can prevent sudden spikes in blood sugar levels.
- **Boosts insulin sensitivity:** Fibre improves the effectiveness of insulin, making it simpler to control blood sugar and manage diabetes successfully.[19]

The Role of Fibre in Weight Loss

Fibre is a crucial component for maintaining a healthy weight:[20]

- **Helps reduce hunger:**
  Fibre takes up more space in the stomach, making you feel full faster and preventing overeating.
- **Encourages slow eating:**
  Any weight loss method is more effective when combined with mindful, slow eating. High-fibre foods like guava, peanuts and chickpeas require more chewing, naturally slowing down your eating speed. This, in turn, reduces calorie intake.

What are 'negative-calorie' foods?

Some foods, like cucumber, celery or lettuce, have 'negative calories'. This means the calories you burn to digest them could be almost the same or sometimes even more than the calories they give you. You would literally be burning calories because of eating more food!

Before you fill your entire grocery cart with cucumbers and celery, here's the truth: no food actually has negative calories. Your body always gets some energy from food. But these veggies are very low in calories, and high in water and fibre, so they fill you up without adding much energy, which can help with weight management.

Fibre and Heart Disease

Let us explore the ways in which fibre lowers heart disease:

Lowering Cholesterol: Foods like oats, legumes and fruits are rich in soluble fibre, which can help lower LDL cholesterol levels in the blood. Reducing cholesterol levels can lead to a lower risk of heart disease.

Blood Pressure Control: A diet abundant in fruits, vegetables and whole grains can help manage blood pressure, a significant risk factor for heart disease.

Reducing Inflammation: Fibre plays a role in decreasing inflammation throughout the body. Since chronic inflammation can heighten the risk of heart disease, a diet high in fibre can be beneficial for heart health.

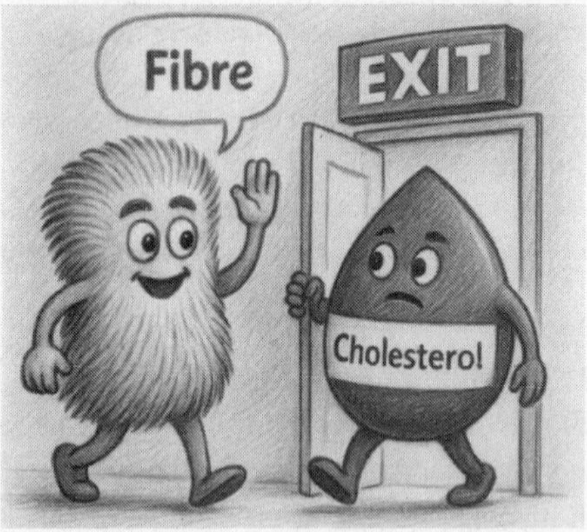

Image 2.8: *Fibre shows cholesterol the exit*

Bottom Line: It is important to aim for at least 30 grams of fibre each day if you are an adult male, and at least 25 grams if you are an adult female.[21] So, how can you reach that 30-gram-fibre goal?

Let's explore the fibre content in the common foods we mentioned earlier.

Food items	**Fibre (in Grams)**
Poha (Breakfast)	1.5 grams
Roti Sabzi (Lunch)	3.5 grams
Vada Pav (with Tea)	3 grams
Dal Rice (Dinner)	4 grams
Total Fibre	**12 grams**

Table 2.1: *Common foods and their fibre content*

Food Item	Fibre (in Grams)	Other Sources of Fibre	Quantity (in Cups)	Fibre (in Grams)	Total Fibre
Poha + Tea (Breakfast)	1.5	Egg + Fruit	1 + 1	4	5.5
Wholewheat Phulka + Sabzi (Lunch)	2.5	Dal + Salad	1.5 Cup + 1 Cup	10	13.5
Tea + Vada Pav (Evening Snacks)	3	Fruit	1	4	7
Rice + Dal (Dinner)	4	Paneer/Chicken + Green Leafy Vegetables	1.5 Cup / 100 Gram + 1 Cup	4	8
Total Fibre	**12**			**22**	**34**

Table 2.2: *Fibre intake through the day*

In a vegetarian diet, fibre intake is generally adequate. However, if we eat as per the above table, which consists of typical meals for most people, it shows that we're only getting 12 grams of fibre. Since our daily fibre requirement is 30 grams, how can we reach this goal?

Let's understand this by making changes to the 'vada pav' sample diet. The aim is to increase the fibre in your diet by making small changes and intentionally incorporating more fibre-rich foods.

To summarise, if we include one fruit at breakfast, a bowl of salad in the afternoon, another fruit in the evening, and some leafy greens for dinner, we can easily surpass 30 grams of fibre. That's all it takes to keep constipation at bay!

Fibre and constipation

Let's be honest, constipation is like Mumbai traffic. Everything is jammed, no one's moving, and you're just sitting there frustrated. Fibre is that smart traffic cop who comes in, clears the mess, and gets things moving again.

Here's how:

1. **Adds volume, like stuffing a beanbag:** Some fibres bulk up your stool, just like stuffing extra beans into a beanbag. That extra volume presses against the walls of your intestine, and your gut gets the signal: 'Arre, time to move!' So, the stool doesn't sit there stuck, it actually moves forward.
2. **Works like a sponge:** Some fibres are total water lovers. They soak up water and turn into a soft gel. Like sabja or chia seeds when you soak them, they puff up and stay moist, holding on to the water. That's exactly what these fibres do to your stool. No more hard, painful lumps, just soft, easy-to-pass poop.
3. **Gives a gentle nudge:** Fibre also physically brushes against your intestinal walls. Your gut responds by releasing a bit of mucus and fluid, and by pushing things along faster.

So, in short, fibre is your gut's broom + wet mop combo. It sweeps, softens and smoothens the whole process. That's why when people eat more sprouts, vegetables, fruits, or even a spoonful of isabgol (psyllium husk), their 'traffic jam' suddenly disappears.

Fibre and acidity: How fibre keeps the fire down

Acidity is like a sudden rush hour in your stomach. Everything's jammed, pressure is building, and things feel out of control. Fibre steps in to bring order.

1. **Holds the gate shut:** It keeps acid from sneaking up where it shouldn't, preventing reflux.
2. **Creates a soft buffer**: It absorbs excess acid and cushions the stomach lining.
3. **Keeps things moving**: It slows stomach movement just enough to avoid sudden acid surges.

In short, fibre is your stomach's traffic controller, keeping everything moving, smooth and calm.

The best part? You don't have to munch on raw veggies to get your fibre fix. Even when you cook vegetables or legumes, the fibre remains intact.

Isn't it a smarter choice to boost your fibre intake this way instead of depending on laxatives and antacids for years? Plus, these fibre-rich foods also offer vital vitamins and minerals. It's a win-win!

How to Increase Fibre in Your Diet?

When someone mentions 'increasing fibre', it doesn't mean you should abruptly switch to a high-fibre diet overnight. Doing so can result in stomach pain, excessive gas, constipation and bloating. There are many cases of people starting on large boluses of chia seeds at random, and then getting bowel obstruction and ending up at the hospital. Dietary fibre, just like any other nutrient, should be increased gradually.

If you've ever swapped rice for millet rotis, and added leafy greens to both lunch and dinner, you may have noticed that your stomach feels heavier than usual. Why does this occur? Because your fibre intake has significantly surged in a short period. A better alternative is to make one change at a time. Instead of white rice, try a millet roti or a multigrain roti. Once you are comfortable with that, add more green veggies or salads. That way, you will not be bloated.

Important: Water is super important when you are increasing your fibre intake. You need to proportionately increase your water intake so that the increase in fibre does not end up giving you hard stool. Otherwise, you might face digestive issues instead of finding relief!

Does fibre get destroyed when making fruit juice?

When fruit is blended or processed in a mixer, the fibre is broken into smaller pieces, but it remains intact. However, blending natural fibre changes how it affects the body.

Our stomach acts like a natural mixer, but it isn't a mechanical blender and can't break down fibre in the same way. Consequently, when you eat a whole fruit, it may take about an hour to digest. In contrast, when the same fruit is consumed as juice, its fibre is broken down or removed (if strained), releasing the sugars, which are quickly absorbed into the bloodstream.

This is why eating whole fruit results in a slow and steady increase in blood sugar levels, while drinking juice can lead to a rapid spike in blood sugar. This difference is mainly due to the breakdown or lack of fibre.

Resistant Starch

Resistant starch has been receiving a lot of attention lately. But what is it really? This type of starch can be found in various foods. For instance, when you steam a potato and allow it to cool, as much as 15 to 50 per cent of its starch can turn into resistant starch.[22]

This means that rather than being absorbed in the stomach and small intestine, this starch makes its way to the colon (large intestine), where it acts as nourishment for beneficial gut bacteria.

If you're looking to boost the resistant starch in your meals, just cook your food and let it chill in the fridge overnight before reheating and eating it the next day. It is this cook-cool-reheat process that increases the resistant starch in starchy foods.

Of course, this doesn't mean you should indulge in endless boiled potatoes or cold rice every day. But for those who love potatoes, this is a fun fact to share in conversations!

We began with protein and then recognized the significance of fibre. Now we understand that vegetables should accompany paneer or chicken. But what about **fat**?

3

Fats

Understanding Fats

When you hear the term 'fat', you might instantly think of body fat. However, fats are more than just what we store in our bodies—they play a crucial role in our diet. In fact, your brain is composed of about 60 per cent fat![1] That's how important fats are to our body.

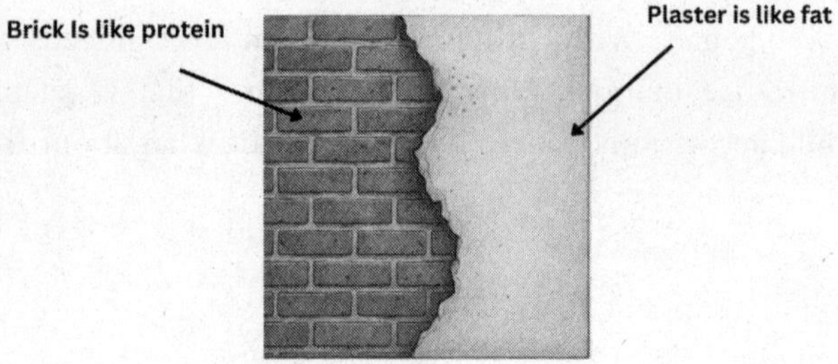

Image 3.1: Plaster is like fat

When I discussed protein, I likened it to a wall. If proteins are 'just another brick in the wall', then fat acts as the cement that binds the bricks in the wall together, ensuring the wall remains strong and resilient.

In our bodies, fat is vital for regulating temperature, storing energy and protecting essential organs. Without fat, the body (the wall) might still stand, but it would be more susceptible—unable to retain heat, lacking shock protection, and having inadequate energy reserves.

This is an important consideration when aiming for fat loss. If body fat levels drop too low, it can result in hormonal imbalances.[2] Fat is crucial for survival, which is why no one should strive for a zero-fat diet, or completely cut out oils, ghee and other healthy fats from their meals.

Importance of Fats in the Human Body

- **Energy Source:** Fats provide long-lasting energy to the body. In fact, the body has only one mechanism for storing excess calories—any extra energy is stored as fat.
- **Cell Structure:** Fats play a crucial role in the structure of every cell in the body. Without fats, cells wouldn't be able to exist. Fats literally make up each cell wall!
- **Hormone Production:** Many hormones in the body are produced using fats. That's why extreme crash diets or zero-oil diets can disrupt hormone balance.
- **Homeostasis and Temperature Regulation:** Dietary fats help regulate body temperature and aid in the absorption of fat-soluble vitamins (A, D, E and K). Body fat also acts as insulation—not just for temperature control but also to protect organs from physical shocks.

Where Do We Get Fats from in Our Diet?

We obtain fats from:

- **Cooking oils, ghee, butter and vanaspati**: These are the fats we use for preparing meals. These are also called 'visible fat'.

- **Naturally occurring fats in foods**: Many foods naturally contain fat, such as milk and dairy products, avocado, almonds, walnuts, sunflower seeds, eggs, chicken, fish, mutton, prawns, crab, etc. This is also known as 'invisible fat'.
- **Hidden fats**: It is found in ultra-processed foods like biscuits, cakes, chips, mayonnaise, bread spread, frozen and ready-to-eat foods, etc.

When discussing fat intake, it's important to consider all three kinds—the naturally occurring fats in foods, the added visible fat, and the hidden fat. However, in most diets, added fats and hidden fats found in packaged foods typically make up the largest portion of total fat intake.

What are hidden fats?

Think of hidden fats as sneaky actors wearing masks. You don't see them directly on your plate like ghee, butter or oil. Instead, they hide inside biscuits, cakes, chips, namkeen, samosas, creamy desserts and packaged foods. You take a bite thinking it's just a light snack, but behind the taste, these invisible fats quietly enter your body. Over time, they pile up in your blood as cholesterol, and around your belly as fat. That's why they are called hidden—because they don't look oily, but they act the same way once inside your body.

Health-washing vs. the health food paradox

Health-washing is a marketing strategy where brands make foods look healthier than they actually are. They do this by using buzzwords like 'organic', 'low-fat', 'multigrain', 'high-protein', or 'sugar-free' on the packaging. While these words sound good, the product may still be high in sugar, refined flour, fat or preservatives.

Example: A biscuit labeled 'multigrain and protein-packed' might still contain refined flour and sugar. The brand is essentially 'dressing up' an unhealthy food in a healthy costume.

The health food paradox is what happens to consumers because of such marketing. People buy foods thinking they are healthy and eat them freely, but end up consuming too many calories, sugar or fats. Over time, this can cause weight gain and reduced health benefits, even though the intention was to eat 'healthy'.

Example: You pick a 'sugar-free' chocolate thinking it's a healthy snack, only to discover it's full of fat and calories. You aimed to eat smart, but the product tricked you—that's the paradox.

How Do Fat Cells Grow When You Eat More Fat?

- **Hypertrophy:** Increase in the size of an individual fat cell.
- **Hyperplasia:** Formation of new fat cells.

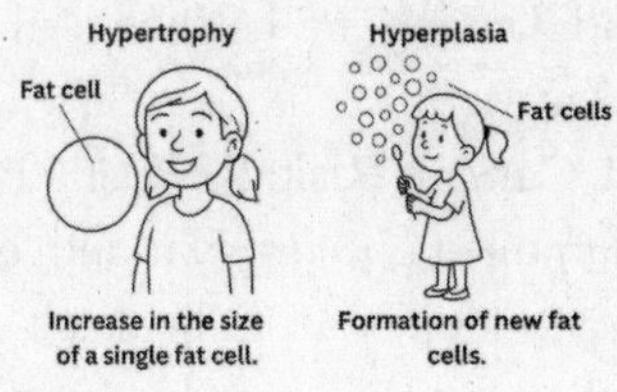

Image 3.2: *How do fat cells grow?*

Important: Once fat cells are created, they stay in the body for life. While their size can change with weight fluctuations, the overall number of fat cells does not decrease.

Some lucky folks who look super slim and seem to have a normal body weight could still have a high body fat percentage and very low muscle mass (skinny fat). If these lucky people eat food that has high quantities of fat, they will eventually find that their bloodwork and health parameters are not as lucky as it seems. When their medical evaluations are conducted, important health indicators such as cholesterol and triglycerides may show imbalances. Consequently, even with a normal weight, they could still face a greater risk of heart disease. This is because lifestyle disorder risk is linked to fat consumption and free fatty acid levels in the body.[3]

Potential Risks of Excessive Oil Consumption

- **Heart Disease and Cardiovascular Issues**: A high intake of fats can contribute to plaque accumulation in the arteries, raising the likelihood of heart disease.[4]
- **Diabetes Risk**: An excessive amount of oil combined with an unhealthy diet can impair insulin function, which may lead to diabetes, even in individuals without a family history.
- **Hormonal Imbalance and Obesity:** A diet rich in fats and lacking in balance can interfere with hormone levels.[5]
- **Increased Cancer Risk**: Regularly consuming more than 1 liter of oil or ghee every month over an extended period may elevate an individual's risk of cancer. Although the effects may not be immediately apparent, they can affect one's health 20–30 years down the line.[67]

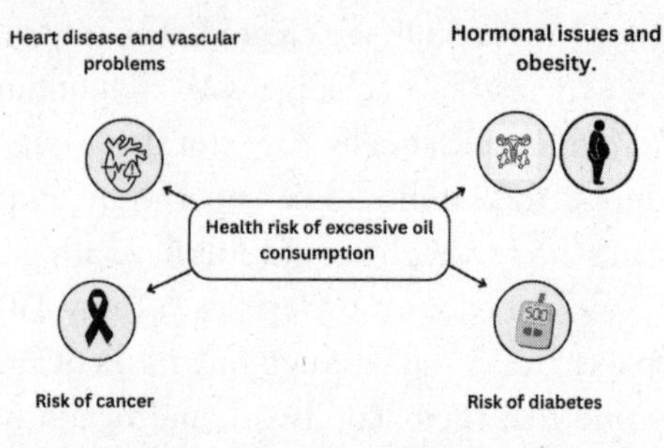

Image 3.3: *Health risks associated with excess oil consumption*

Recommended Fat Intake as per ICMR and NIN Guidelines

According to the Indian Council of Medical Research (ICMR) and the National Institute of Nutrition (NIN) guidelines, an individual should consume 25–30 grams (approximately 5 teaspoons) of fats daily, including oil, ghee and butter.

How much is 25–30 grams?

Remember, 1 teaspoon of oil is approximately 5 grams, so 25–30 grams amounts to 5–6 teaspoons of oil, ghee or butter per day. Do note: it is teaspoons and not tablespoons.

Measuring oil or ghee for a family

- To calculate oil usage for the entire family, each person's total monthly oil and ghee intake should not exceed 750 ml.
- For example, in a family of four, monthly oil consumption should not exceed 2 litres, and ghee should be limited to 1 litre for the whole family.

Excessive oil and ghee intake can lead to obesity, heart disease, high blood pressure and digestive issues. This calculation assumes that, along with oil, you are also consuming ghee, butter, packaged foods and other fat sources.

Note: If your hidden fat consumption due to ultra-processed foods is too high, then you will need to significantly reduce your added fat intake, otherwise you will end up taking in too much fat each day.

Fat-free or oil-free diet

Oil or ghee-free diets have become quite popular these days. People often follow them to lose weight or control blood sugar, thinking that avoiding fat will help. However, there is no scientific basis to this approach. Fat is extremely important for the body. Following a fat-free diet can lead to hormonal imbalances and can negatively affect the health of your muscles, nervous system and heart.

Fat is not bad; it is essential. The key is simply to maintain the right amount of fat in your diet.

Understanding Added Fats

Now, let's take a closer look at cooking oils, ghee, butter and vanaspati, which consist of specific types of fatty acids. The following table outlines the fatty acid composition in various oils.

Types of Fat	Health Impact	Sources
Saturated Fats	Excessive consumption can increase cholesterol levels and raise the risk of heart disease.	Ghee, butter, coconut oil, palm oil, full-fat dairy products
Monounsaturated Fats (Healthy Fats)	They are beneficial for the heart, reduce bad cholesterol (LDL), and help maintain good cholesterol (HDL).	Olive oil, peanut oil, sesame oil, mustard oil, rice bran oil, sunflower oil, avocado, almonds
Polyunsaturated Fats (Healthy Fats)	Essential fatty acids like Omega-3 and Omega-6 are important for brain function and heart health. They help reduce bad cholesterol (LDL).	Sunflower oil, soybean oil, sesame, flaxseeds, walnuts, fish (mackerel, sardines), chia seeds
Avoid Trans Fats (Unhealthy Fats)	Found in processed and junk foods, it increases bad cholesterol (LDL) and reduces good cholesterol (HDL).	Packaged snacks, deep-fried foods, bakery items and vanaspati

Table 3.1: *Type of fats*

Different oils should be consumed as a part of one's diet. The total amount of fat should be kept to 5–6 teaspoons per day. For example, if you use peanut oil to cook vegetables in the morning and evening, you can add some ghee to the salad or dal to ensure a varied fatty acid profile in your meals.

Which Oil to Use, and Which Oil Is Good?

Different oils are suited for different dishes. Just like we consume a variety of vegetables, we obtain distinct nutrients from various oils. It's best to choose oils that are rich in MUFA (monounsaturated fatty acids), which is why olive oil is a favourite.[8] But it's not necessary to limit oneself to fancy imported oils. We can also support our health by using traditional Indian regional oils in appropriate amounts.

PUFA	MUFA	SFA
Mustard oil, groundnut (peanut) oil, rice bran oil, sunflower oil, safflower oil, sesame oil	Sesame oil, sunflower oil, soybean oil, olive oil	Coconut oil

Table 3.2: *Oils to use*

Fatty Acids from Oils: What are PUFA, MUFA and SFA?

We often see these fancy terms—PUFA, MUFA and SFA—on oil bottles or health articles. These are nothing but the smaller fatty acids that make up these oils.

MUFA (monounsaturated fats): Oils high in MUFA are generally the good guys for your heart.[9] MUFA-rich oils help the heart run smoothly. Think olive oil, mustard oil, peanut oil—these keep your cholesterol in check when used in the right amount.

SFA (saturated fats): Oils or fats high in SFA include coconut oil, butter, ghee, lard, tallow or, the worst offender of all, hydrogenated vegetable oils (like vanaspati). These can increase your bad cholesterol (LDL) if you overdo them.[10,11] So the golden rule is: two teaspoons, fine. Beyond that? Please put the spoon down!

Excess SFA means higher chances of clogged arteries—not exactly what you want. That's why hydrogenated oils are a big *no*.[12]

So, what's the smart way? **Rotate your oils!** Don't stick to just one oil forever. Use olive oil for a month, switch to rice bran oil the next month, then maybe mustard oil. This way, your body gets a healthy mix of fatty acids, and your taste buds won't complain either.

Bottomline: variety and moderation are key.

Speaking of variety, if you are like me and like to eat something other than the standard roti-sabzi or dal-rice for dinner, then this list is going to be helpful for you. Suitable oils for different types of dishes:

- Asian or Thai food: Sesame oil
- Mediterranean food: Olive oil
- Chinese food: Soybean oil, rapeseed oil
- Sri Lankan food: Coconut oil, peanut oil
- North Indian and/or Punjabi dishes: Mustard oil
- South Indian dishes like sambar, idli, dosa, etc.: Coconut oil
- Maharashtrian, Gujarati, Rajasthani dishes: Peanut oil

Mixed seeds

These days, mixed seeds are quite popular as a healthy snack or a source of good fats. And yes—they *are* healthy, but are also a source of fats and are pretty high in calories.

Here's what people forget: if you overeat them, they can still lead to weight gain, increase your cholesterol, give you acidity and reflux, and even put extra strain on your digestion due to high amounts of insoluble fibre.

So, don't go overboard. About **2 tablespoons a day** is more than enough. No need to pour seeds from a packet on every meal you have and call it 'healthy eating'. As always, balance is key!

How Many Nuts Should You Really Eat? And What About Peanuts?

Most of us can safely enjoy a *small handful* of nuts daily. But then the question pops up: what about peanuts? And why do some people get pimples after eating almonds?

Here's the simple truth: nuts are healthy, but they're also heavy on digestion. Cashews, pistachios, almonds, peanuts—all of these nuts are about **50 per cent fat**. So, if till yesterday you barely ate any nuts, and today you start eating an entire handful every day all of a sudden, your body might protest. What happens then? Indigestion, breakouts, bloating or stomach pain—all pretty common. Why? Because nuts don't just contain healthy fats; they also pack in fibre. Nuts contain a good amount of fibre, which can also become difficult to digest for those particularly sensitive to sudden large quantities of fibre.

And for some people, this fibre can be tough to digest at first, which shows up as pimples or stomach trouble.

So, remember this golden rule: whenever you start eating something new, especially nuts, **start small**. Give your stomach time to adjust, then gradually increase the amount. Your skin and tummy will thank you later!

Refined Oil vs. Cold-Pressed Oil

If you browse social media today, you might get the impression that using refined oil is a major health mistake. There's a lot of talk about switching to cold-pressed oil, but that perspective isn't completely accurate. Let me try to explain this to you with an analogy. When I want to run an errand at the local shop, I can either walk or use a two-wheeler, and I'll get there quickly. However, if I opt for a large, expensive vehicle, the cost of that trip will be unnecessarily and significantly higher.

If you're planning to deep fry something, using a high-quality oil like extra virgin or cold-pressed oil isn't the best choice. These oils are less processed and retain vitamins A, E and K because they haven't been exposed to high heat. However, when you use them for frying, those nutrients get destroyed. That's why refined oils are better suited for frying. Cold-pressed oils can spoil quickly and might alter the flavour of certain dishes. While coconut oil and mustard oil have high smoke points and are suitable for frying, I still wouldn't recommend using cold-pressed variants of those oils for deep frying.

You might have noticed the phrase 'added vitamins' on the labels of refined oils. This is because the refining process involves heating the oil to high temperatures, which destroys the natural vitamins. As a result, these vitamins need to be reintroduced in a chemical form, which is why you see 'added vitamins' on the packaging.

Another key point regarding refined oils has to do with the 'cholesterol free' label. Does it mean that your cholesterol levels will not increase if you consume these oils that are labelled as such?

Cholesterol is only found in animal-based products like butter, ghee and meat. It is not naturally present in plant-based products such as oils. However, that doesn't mean that oil can't affect the cholesterol levels in the body. When fatty acids from oil are consumed in large quantities, the body can produce cholesterol on its own. So, even though oil doesn't contain cholesterol, consuming it in excess can still lead to increased cholesterol levels.[13]

Cold-pressed oils are free from solvents and undergo minimal processing. They can be used for daily cooking, but they are not suitable for deep frying. For deep frying, it's better to use refined oils. Cold-pressed oils work well for cooking vegetables, dals or parathas.

It's important to remember that just because cold-pressed or unrefined oils have more micronutrients, doesn't mean you should consume them in large quantities. After all, they are still oils. **Excessive consumption of even cold-pressed or unrefined oils can contribute to heart blockages.**

Extra-virgin and cold-pressed oils are essentially the same. To use them correctly, they should be enjoyed in their raw form-like drizzled on chutneys or as salad dressings.

Keep this guideline in mind:

- Extra-virgin, cold-pressed and unrefined oils: For raw consumption or everyday cooking, sautéing or quick cooking like in sabzis and stir fries.
- Refined oils: For deep frying

By adhering to this, you'll ensure the oil is used properly, benefiting your health. However, it's important to remember that even with cold-pressed oil, moderation is key.

'Do I only have to use cold-pressed or extra-virgin oil? It is too expensive!' I agree. While a cold-pressed oil with a better MUFA to PUFA ratio, like olive oil kardi oil, is better and almost ideal, it is not something that everyone can afford for every meal, especially considering that we are often cooking for more than one person at a time. Here's the real deal: like I have already mentioned before, just because it is extra-virgin, it does not mean that it can be consumed in unlimited amounts. The corollary is also true! Even if you are only using refined oil, fitting your budget and limiting the quantity of that oil to 5 teaspoons a day as we explained earlier, you will be in better shape than someone who is consuming 10 tablespoons of extra-virgin olive oil. This is simply because the sheer amount of daily oil consumption is a bigger risk factor for your health than which seed oil you use.[14,15] (Palm oil and coconut oil are exceptions here as they are mostly saturated fat.)

If it's not within your budget, opting for refined oil is also okay;[16] **what's truly important is the amount of oil you consume!**

How to Keep Control over Oil Use?

- Instead of pouring oil, measure it using a spoon.
- You can also try applying oil with a brush instead of drizzling it on food.
- Opt for baking, steaming or boiling instead of frying.

- While cooking, add a drop of water to help cook with less oil.
- Keep track of your monthly oil consumption and ensure it does not exceed 750 ml per person.

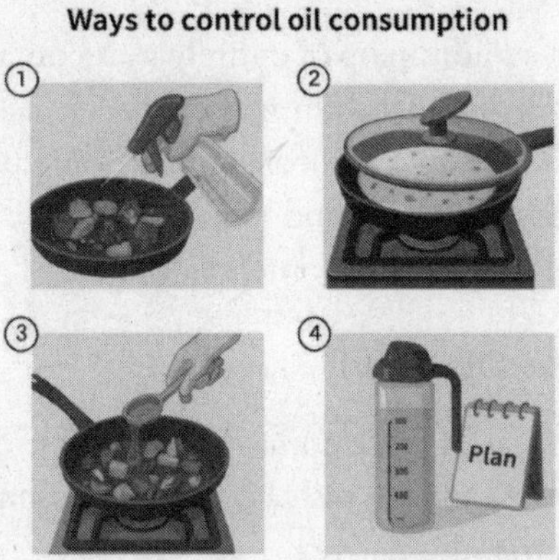

Image 3.4: *Ways to control oil consumption*

How to Incorporate Different Oils in Our Diet?

Using various types of oils can be challenging for some, especially if small bottles are hard to find or are too pricey. If you face this issue, consider trying the rotation method. For instance:

- Use peanut oil this month.
- Switch to mustard oil next month.
- Then use safflower oil the month after that.

This approach allows you to enjoy the benefits of different kinds of fatty acids.

Cottonseed Oil and Palm Oil: Common in Hotels but Unhealthy

These oils are high in saturated fat. Palm oil has 52 per cent saturated fatty acids (SFA), while cottonseed oil contains 24 per cent SFA.

It's best to avoid vanaspati entirely as it contains trans fats that can be detrimental to heart health.[17]

You may already be consuming vanaspati through biscuits, packaged snacks and namkeen at home, so there's no need to use it in your home cooking.

How to Use Olive Oil?

- Steer clear of olive pomace oil as it is produced from leftover residue.[18] Instead, consider using peanut oil as a better alternative.
- Reserve extra-virgin olive oil for salads and stir-fries only.

Can We Reuse Oil Used for Deep Frying?

A common question, and an important one!

First things first, please *don't* heat up a huge kadhai full of oil for frying just because it feels convenient. Sure, it might save you some time now, but here's what usually happens—you don't end up using all that oil in one go, and then you feel guilty about wasting it, or you keep reusing it for days.

Instead, do this, use a *smaller* kadhai and fry in smaller batches. Yes, it might take a few extra minutes, but you'll use less oil, and you won't feel bad about leftover oil lying around.

Why is this important? Because each time you reheat the same oil, it gets chemically altered—forming *trans fats*.

Even if you're using so-called 'clean' or expensive oils, once you heat them repeatedly, they're not so healthy anymore.

So, here's the smart way:

- Fry in small batches.
- Don't eat deep-fried food every day (your arteries will thank you).
- Don't store used frying oil for weeks.

If you do have leftover oil after frying, strain it immediately while it's warm, and *use it up within the next two days*, maybe for cooking veggies. Don't hoard used oil for a week. Once heated, the unsaturated fats start turning into saturated or even trans fats, which are bad news for your health.

Small tweaks, big health wins, and zero guilt about wasted oil. Fry smart!

Coconut and coconut oil

What happens if you eat too much coconut?

Excess consumption of coconut can lead to weight gain, as it is a source of fat in the form of medium-chain triglycerides (MCTs) and saturated fats. This may increase cholesterol and triglyceride levels. While coconut is healthy, it should be consumed in moderation.[19]

How much coconut oil is appropriate?

When it comes to coconut oil, 2–3 teaspoons per day is a good limit. Coconut oil can be used as a substitute for ghee, but the intake of excess saturated fat should be avoided. Do not cook everything in coconut oil daily; use a variety of oils instead.

Does coconut help in weight loss?

Coconut may help slightly as it contains fat and fibre, which can keep you full for longer. However, consuming it in large amounts daily can lead to weight gain.

Does drinking coconut water help in weight loss?
Coconut water does not directly help in weight loss, but it is great for hydration. It does not significantly reduce calorie intake, but it helps maintain the body's electrolyte balance.

Is coconut milk healthy?
Coconut milk is a good vegan option, but it is high in fat. If you have cholesterol or triglyceride issues, its consumption should be limited.

How to include coconut in your daily diet?
You can add fresh grated coconut to vegetables, poha, dailya and other dishes. Two tablespoons of fresh coconut per day is a good amount, but avoid excessive intake.

Is Ghee Healthy?

Yes, ghee is indeed healthy! There's nothing inherently unhealthy about it. However, it's essential to keep in mind that ghee is a type of fat, similar to oil or butter, which provides necessary fats for the body. Therefore, just as we use oil or butter in moderation, ghee should also be consumed in controlled amounts.

The key to balance is maintaining a 2:1:1 ratio among PUFA, MUFA and SFA. Ghee is categorised as a saturated fat, much like butter. Butter and coconut oil are also primarily made up of saturated fats.

For daily intake, a person should aim for about 25–30 grams of added fat (fat consumed separately from food). If someone consumes around 5 teaspoons of fat each day, then 1 to 2 teaspoons of ghee is a reasonable amount.

Does Eating Too Much Ghee Lead to Weight Gain?

Yes, absolutely! The more fat you consume, the more fat your body stores.

Cow ghee vs. buffalo ghee

The claim that 'buffalo ghee causes weight gain, but cow ghee burns fat' is just a marketing gimmick.

Both types of ghee are fats and have a similar calorie content. Weight gain or fat loss does not depend on the type of ghee you consume, but rather on how much ghee you consume. The same is true for A1 or A2 ghee; nutritionally, both are the same.

Ghee is pure fat, meaning it only provides fatty acids and very few other nutrients. It does contain some vitamin D, but in negligible amounts. So, relying on ghee for vitamin D is not a good idea. It's better to eat eggs or sun-exposed mushrooms instead!

One teaspoon of ghee contains 9 calories per gram. If you don't measure how much ghee you're eating, hidden calories can add up, increasing the risk of weight gain.

Besides weight gain, excess ghee can also raise cholesterol levels. Cholesterol and triglycerides don't shoot up overnight, but regularly eating too much ghee can cause them to increase over time.[20]

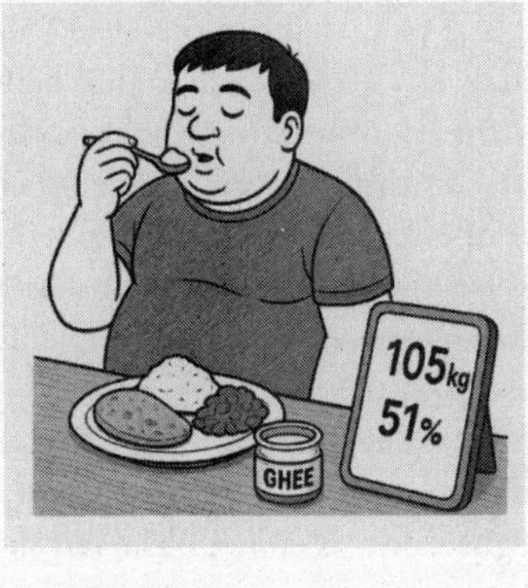

Image 3.5: *Ghee and weight gain*

A1 vs. A2 milk: Which one is actually better?

A1 and A2 refer to types of proteins found in milk. A1 milk contains a peptide called BCM-7, which, in some studies, has been linked to increased insulin resistance. However, these studies were limited, and there is no solid scientific proof that A1 milk is harmful. When it comes to ghee, it is a pure fat and does not contain any proteins including any BCM-7. Since all proteins are completely removed during the process of making ghee, A1 or A2 has nothing to do with ghee!

'A2 ghee' is just a marketing gimmick. Whether it's cow ghee or buffalo ghee, what matters is how much of it you consume. There's no need to spend extra money on A2 ghee in the hopes of it giving you any extra health benefits. Even A2, bilona and organic farm ghee can clog your arteries and trouble your heart!

Ghee vs. oil: What's the real difference?

Ghee and oil are not the same when it comes to the kind of fats they give us.

- Ghee mainly gives us saturated fats.
- Oils (like groundnut, sunflower, rice bran, mustard) give us healthy MUFA and PUFA.

In fact, research shows that the more seed oils you consume, replacing saturated fat in your diet, the better your health outcomes.[21] This does not mean that you start drinking seed oils, but out of the total fat that you consume, it is better for the ratio to skew in favour of oils instead of ghee or butter.

For our body to stay healthy, all these fats need to stay in balance, like a team where everyone has a role. The ideal ratio is PUFA:MUFA:SFA = 2:1:1.

So, if your daily fat allowance is about 25 grams, only a small share should come from ghee. In practical terms, that means just 1–2 teaspoons of ghee a day is enough. The rest should come from different oils.

Which Is Better: Store-Bought or Homemade Ghee?

When purchasing ghee, it's important to think about the production process. Fermentation significantly influences the fatty acid profile of ghee, and the quality of store-bought options largely depends on their manufacturing methods.

Homemade ghee offers a unique taste and aroma since it is typically made from cultured butter. You can source butter from a local dairy, add some starter curd culture to it, keep it overnight and then make ghee in your own kitchen. Of course, the best option is following the traditional method of storing cream from milk every day, and then making culture butter from it, which in turn is boiled to make ghee.

When choosing packaged ghee, pay attention to its taste, colour and production method. Homemade ghee usually has a deeper colour and a stronger aroma, while store-bought ghee is generally lighter and milder in flavour. Thus, evaluating the quality of ghee requires careful consideration of its taste and preparation method.

Vanaspati is not ghee, it's actually oil!

No, they are not the same at all!

Vegetable oil, including palm oil, is derived from various plants, and is typically a refined product. Many biscuits, snacks and ready-to-eat foods you find in stores often contain 'refined vegetable oil', which is not ghee.

The difference?

Ghee is natural and free from trans fats when prepared properly.

Vegetable oil (and vanaspati) may contain harmful trans fats that can hurt your heart and overall health.

What most people call vanaspati ghee isn't ghee at all; it's hydrogenated vegetable oil, chemically processed and solidified to look like ghee.[2]

Is It Right to Only Rely on Ghee for All Our Cooking?

Our body needs various fatty acids as explained in the tables above (3.1 and 3.2). If we use only ghee for all our cooking, we will end up significantly skewing the fatty acid ratios in favour of too much saturated fat. We know that high saturated fat intake leads to high cholesterol levels and increases our risk of lifestyle disorders. Hence, it is always advisable to use a combination of oil and ghee in our cooking.

Why Is It Popular to Consume Ghee with Warm Water in the Morning?

In our parents' generation, people used to drink milk with ghee at night, or ghee with warm water in the morning. This was mainly done for constipation relief (to ensure smooth bowel movements). Since ghee acts as a natural lubricant, it helps in elimination.

Can People Who Do Not Drink Milk or Cannot Digest It Still Consume Ghee?

Yes, people with lactose intolerance who cannot digest milk, yogurt or paneer can still consume ghee.

Lactose is a type of sugar, whereas ghee is pure fat. Ghee is boiled at such a high temperature that all the lactose and milk proteins (casein) separate and settle at the bottom. What remains on top is pure fat.

That's why even those who cannot digest milk can safely consume ghee as it does not contain any lactose!

Biscuits and fats?

Store-bought biscuits should be avoided because they contain vanaspati (hydrogenated fat). The real problem with biscuits is overconsumption and habit formation. They easily become a part of our daily diet—whether with tea or as a quick snack when feeling slightly hungry. Especially wafer biscuits—they seem light but actually have as much fat as if they were deep-fried, and some contain even more fat than puris made with ghee!

Instead of grabbing a biscuit whenever hunger strikes, it's always better to keep healthier snacks ready in advance. There are plenty of alternatives to biscuits. You just need to be willing to change the habit!

You might ask, what if I make biscuits at home using whole wheat flour, ghee and jaggery. Can I eat homemade biscuits every day?

Even if a biscuit or cookie is made at home using millet, ragi, ghee or jaggery, it still remains a product that is high in refined ingredients. Usually, these recipes call for around 50–70 per cent flour, 15–35 per cent fat, and 10–25 per cent sugar. Whether you bake them yourself or grab them from a so-called 'healthy' brand, they still add extra fat and sugar to your diet, essentially empty calories that our bodies don't really need. This goes for both adults and kids. So, if your child occasionally asks for a biscuit or cookie, feel free to offer a homemade or millet-based one, but keep it in moderation. It's crucial to remember that biscuits, cookies or rusks, no matter how wholesome they claim to be, shouldn't become a daily snack. They should stay an occasional treat, not a dietary habit.

If biscuits are not okay, can we have toast and khari instead?

Toast looks dry, which makes it seem 'light', but check its nutrition label—it contains 33.18 per cent fat! It is extra saturated fat that we don't need! Also, what is this obsession with eating something with tea?

What about cream biscuits?

Cream biscuits contain more than 50 per cent fat, and the 'cream' you eat is not real cream—it's just a paste made of vanaspati (hydrogenated fat) and sugar! If real ghee were used, it would melt, but vanaspati remains solid at room temperature, and hence gets used in sugar-cream-filled biscuits.

We apply pure ghee on rotis for our kids, yet we feed them biscuits made with vanaspati. Does that seem like the right choice to you?

Fatty Liver and Fat

Fatty liver is a condition often linked to lifestyle choices, and it can be effectively managed through proper diet and lifestyle adjustments.

Saturated fat is prevalent in foods like ghee, butter, dairy products and red meat. For instance, mutton contains such high levels of saturated fat that it can account for an entire day's worth of fat intake. Hence, people with fatty liver should limit their intake of red meat and foods high in saturated fats.[23]

From a health standpoint, adults should aim to consume no more than two teaspoons of saturated fat daily. Moreover, even healthier fats found in almonds, walnuts and peanuts should be eaten in moderation. Just because a food is labeled as 'healthy' doesn't mean it can be consumed without limits; eating too much can also contribute to excess fat buildup in the body.

Thus, it's crucial to maintain a balanced intake of oils, ghee, nuts and other fats.

Visceral fat, subcutaneous fat and abdominal fat

What is visceral fat?

Think of it like bubble wrap—except instead of covering us externally, this fatty bubble wrap wraps itself around your internal organs. If your diet is high in fat or you have excess body fat in general, this internal layer builds up quietly around your vital organs. It's sneaky, and it can cause health troubles if it gets too thick.

What is subcutaneous fat?

It is the fat that sits *just under your skin.* This is the soft layer you can pinch, like belly fat or the bit under your arms. This fat actually plays an important role: it helps regulate your body temperature, cushions your organs from bumps and knocks, and provides some basic protection.

What is abdominal fat?

It is simply the fat stored around your stomach area, and it includes *both* subcutaneous and visceral fat. So, when we talk about 'belly fat', we're really talking about this combo.

Keeping visceral fat in check is especially important for good health, so balanced food, regular movement, and not overdoing processed fats is the way to go. Your organs will thank you for it!

Do People with Diabetes Also Need to Be Careful About Their Fat Intake?

For individuals with diabetes, managing sugar intake is certainly important, but monitoring fat consumption is equally essential.[24] Effective diabetes management involves balancing sugar and carbohydrate intake while also including healthy fats. This can be achieved by incorporating foods like almonds, walnuts and extra-virgin olive oil.

It's important to keep an eye on the amount of fat consumed, particularly for those with diabetes. Aim to limit your fat intake to no more than 25 grams per day, as consuming too much fat can elevate the risk of heart problems and other diabetes-related complications.[25]

Does Eating Oily Food Cause Acne or Pimples?

An unhealthy diet can manifest in various ways in your body. Some individuals may develop acne, while others might face digestive issues like loose motions or constipation—sometimes going days without a bowel movement or having difficulty when they do. Common symptoms also include stomach pain and acidity. These are all indicators that something in your diet and gut needs attention.

When digestion is off, it can lead to skin problems. Eating too many oily and greasy foods can exacerbate these issues. Teenagers, particularly those aged 13 to 19, are especially prone to pimples due to their often-irregular eating habits and hormonal fluctuations. Teenagers and young adults are also prone to not eating enough fibre, which also contributes to the ravages of adolescence, in this case, acne.

Consuming excessive oil can lead to a higher calorie intake, so cutting back on oil can be beneficial to some degree. However, it's important to note that pimples aren't solely caused by oily foods.

Top Tips to Manage Fat in Your Diet

1. Avoid fried foods whenever possible. Occasionally eating something like puri, papad or jalebi during festivals is fine, but avoid making it a regular habit.
2. Be careful when eating out. Most restaurant foods are usually cooked in hydrogenated vegetable oils—high in fat and loaded with trans fats. Better to opt for grilled or tandoor options instead of deep-fried.
3. Check nutrition labels even for baked goods. Just because something is baked doesn't always mean it's low in fat. Always compare and verify the total fat content.
4. Get healthy fats from nuts. Almonds, walnuts, pistachios, peanuts and cashews are excellent sources. You can have a handful in the morning or as a snack in the afternoon,

but not with tea or coffee (why you should not have it with tea or coffee is something you will learn in the chapter on micronutrients).

5. Add a small amount of healthy fat to meals. One tablespoon of nut or seed chutney (like sesame, flax or peanut) can be included in each meal.
6. Control cooking oil at home. Take oil in a small container and use just a teaspoon at a time to better estimate how much you're using. A person typically needs only 5–6 teaspoons of oil and 1–1.5 teaspoons of ghee per day. Using oil straight from a big container makes it hard to track.
7. Avoid packaged bakery items and snacks. Biscuits, toast, khari, nankhatai, jeera butter—these are all high in hydrogenated vegetable oils and offer almost no nutritional value.
8. Use an air fryer. It's a great appliance to make crunchy snacks without deep frying.
9. Don't reuse frying oil. If you have leftover oil from frying, use it for sautéing vegetables instead, to prevent the formation of trans fats.
10. Watch for excess oil in curries and dals. If oil is visibly floating or pooling on top, it likely comes from fatty ingredients and adds unnecessary fat.

Feeling confident about the role of fat and how much we need to eat it? Next, let's turn our attention to **rotis and rice.**

4
Carbohydrates

Protein builds the walls or structure of the body, and fibre sets up a kind of software system to help it function. But to actually get things running, you need fuel. That fuel is carbohydrates, or carbs. Carbohydrates are an essential nutrient that provides energy to our body. They're especially important for our day-to-day activities and for our brain to function properly. That's why, when we're hungry and say things like 'My brain just isn't working right now', it's usually because our carb levels—or energy—are low. When we feel restless, weak or even a bit sleepy when we're hungry, that's our body's way of asking for energy too.

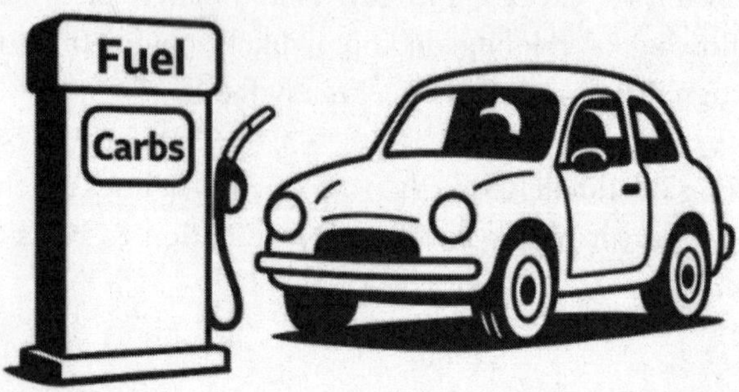

Image 4.1: *Carbohydrates: the body's primary fuel*

Carbs also play a big role in that feeling of satisfaction we get after a meal. Ever wonder why eating rice at night feels like a 'complete meal'? That's because the reward centre in our brain lights up when we eat carbs and protein—it makes us feel content. In fact, if there were a currency the body uses to finance all its functions, it would be carbs.

Our body performs about 37 thousand billion chemical reactions every second, and carbs—in some form—are involved in 99 per cent of them. And that's not all. The brain's primary and most important fuel is also a type of carbohydrate: glucose.

Despite being so essential, carbs are often unfairly blamed. People say things like 'rice makes you fat', 'sweets cause diabetes', or 'eating maida leads to weight gain'. Some even believe that completely cutting out carbs completely is the only way to lose weight. But the truth is, none of this is entirely accurate.

We'll dive deeper into the *why* soon, but here's something to keep in mind: carbs are a crucial macronutrient. If you eliminate them entirely from your diet, it becomes very hard to stay healthy in the long run. After all, even our DNA—our very genes—contains a sugar molecule called ribose.[1] **So if our genetic code itself is built on sugar, how can we expect to thrive by completely cutting out carbs?**

Carbohydrates are of two types: simple carbohydrates and complex carbohydrates.

Simple Carbohydrates

Simple carbohydrates get digested quickly and give an instant burst of energy. But just like everything else that works instantly, this energy does not last long. As a result, blood sugar levels can rise and fall quickly.

Sources: white sugar, jaggery, khaand sugar, kakvi, honey, maltose, corn syrup, liquid glucose, palm sugar, coconut sugar, etc.

Complex Carbohydrates

Complex carbohydrates are basically simple sugars trapped in a web of fibre. Because they are locked in, they take longer to digest. Our digestive system has to work harder to extract that energy from within the fibre mesh. In the process of breaking down the complex carbohydrates, our body actually uses up some of the simple sugar that is already in the blood.[2]

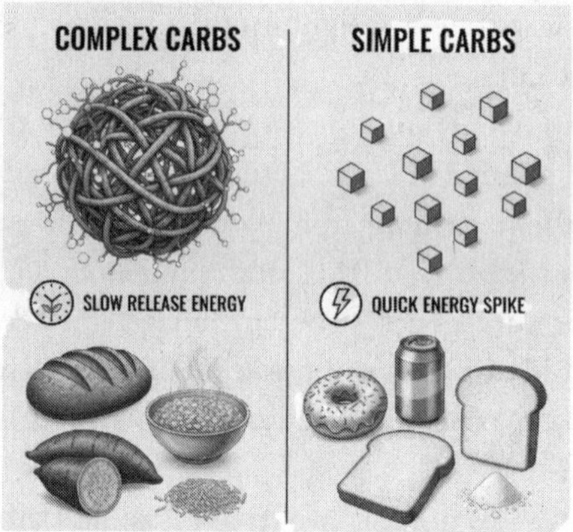

Image 4.2: *Complex and simple carbohydrates*

Since fibre tightly holds on to those sugars, the energy is released slowly and steadily, giving us long-lasting fuel, and helping maintain stable blood sugar levels.

- **Sources**

  Grains: rice, wheat, jowar, bajra

  Legumes: lentils, chickpeas, moong

  Roots and tubers: boiled or roasted potatoes and similar vegetables

  Fruits and vegetables: banana, apple, orange, spinach, carrot

Complex carbohydrates take longer to digest, which is why they help keep you feeling fuller for longer. Do you remember what we discussed about fibre earlier? Since complex carbs contain both simple sugars and fibre, they provide a sense of fullness after a meal and help prevent constant hunger. The presence of fibre also lowers the glycemic index of these foods, meaning they don't cause your blood sugar to spike quickly. This makes complex carbs a much better option for steady energy and blood sugar control.

Sources of Complex Carbohydrates		
White rice	Red rice	Wheat vermicelli
Poha (Flattened rice)	Maida (Refined flour)	Little millet
Rava (Semolina)	Finger millet	Sorghum
Wheat daliya (Cracked wheat)	Little millet	Wheat flour
Amaranth (Rajgira)	Barley	Pearl millet
Wheat	Rice puffed	Sweet corn
Quinoa	Kodo millet (varagu)	

Table 4.1: *Sources of carbohydrates*

Does eating sweets cause diabetes?

Eating sweets does not cause diabetes per se, but having too many sugary drinks, desserts, ultra-processed foods with hidden sugars, homemade jaggery or sweets, loaded snacks, chocolates, jams, chocolate spreads, biscuits, and so on can lead to an overall caloric excess. This caloric excess and high load of 'empty calories' is what leads to type 2 diabetes.

If calorie intake consistently exceeds what the body needs, it can lead to weight gain. When people cut down sugar to lose weight, what they're really doing is reducing their overall calorie intake. And since excess weight is a major risk factor for diabetes,[3] it makes sense to limit sugar wherever possible.

Aren't All Carbohydrates Just 'Sugar' in the End?

At a basic level, yes, most of the carbohydrates we eat eventually get broken down into glucose during digestion. So, it's natural to think that no matter what you eat—rice, wheat, jowar, bajra or even sugar—it all ends up as glucose.

But from a nutrition perspective, is wheat the same as sugar? Not at all.

While sugar is only a 'simple carb', there is no other nutrient in it. But wheat, rice and oats don't just give you glucose or energy. They also provide many important nutrients like whole carbs, fibre, some protein, and some vitamins and minerals. These whole grains contain up to 10 to 15 per cent fibre, which our body cannot digest, but which works as food for our gut microbiome. Grains also contain about 10–12 per cent protein,[4] and of course, other vitamins and minerals like B-complex vitamins and iron, magnesium, phosphorus, zinc and selenium. Because whole carbs are a complex package of nutrition, along with simple sugars or simple carbs, they cannot be compared with derivatives like white sugar.

So, What's the Difference Between Rice, Wheat and Sugar?

Apart from the nutrient profile, even the way these foods are digested in our body varies significantly. When table sugar enters our body, it gets digested quickly, causing a rapid spike in blood sugar (glucose) levels. But wheat and other whole grains contain fibre and protein, which slow down the absorption of glucose.[5] This is why wheat or other grains take longer to digest, and provide a steady, controlled release of energy.

Have you ever eaten raw wheat? I hope not, because it's hard to digest and causes a tummy ache. Whole grains need to be milled and cooked for us to be able to digest them; the same applies to pulses as well. The fibre and other components in whole grains form a structure that prevents them from breaking down too quickly, so they don't cause a rapid rise in blood sugar like table sugar does.

'But Amita, we eat bread, noodles, pasta and pizza. What type of carbs are those?'

These foods are typically made from refined wheat flour, which is maida. Apart from the simple carbs and a bit of protein in wheat, maida doesn't have much nutritional value. That's why foods made from maida are classified as simple, easy-to-digest carbs. Many ultra-processed foods contain only simple carbs and fats, leaving behind most other nutrients.

When we consume such foods, the sugar in our blood rises quickly. If this continues for a long time, it increases the likelihood of developing pre-diabetes or insulin resistance. If someone already has diabetes, consuming high-calorie foods made from maida becomes even more challenging for managing blood glucose levels. While we are on the topic of blood glucose levels and carbohydrates, let's also understand two other terms associated with blood glucose spikes: glycemic index and glycemic load.

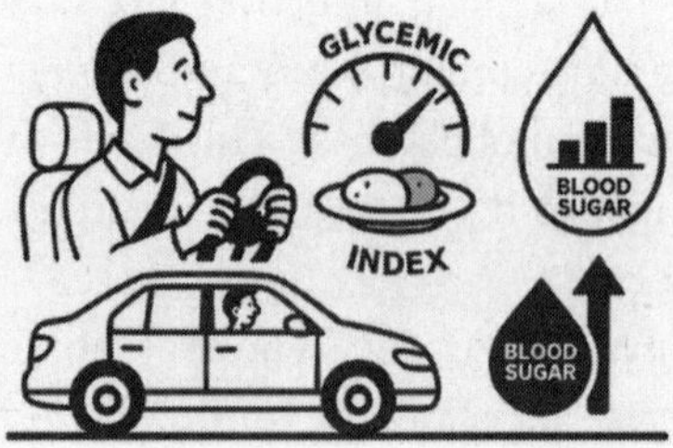

Image 4.3: *Glycemic load*

What is Glycemic Index (GI) and Glycemic Load (GL)?[6,7]

Imagine that you're driving a car; you can tell the speed of the car by looking at the speedometer, right? Similarly, the rate at which your glucose levels increase from the food you eat can be understood by looking at the glycemic index of the food. The higher the glycemic index, the faster your blood glucose or sugar level rises.

An odometer in a car tells you how far the car has gone at a particular speed. Just like that, glycemic load tells you how much or how far the blood sugar level rises based on the glycemic index. Instead of just looking at how fast the blood sugar level rises, it is more important to observe how long the sugar remains elevated, and how much it increases. Just like a car takes longer to return to its starting point the farther it goes, the more your blood sugar rises, the longer it stays elevated, which increases your glycosylated hemoglobin. HbA1C is the most important test to see whether diabetes is being properly managed or not.

So, as explained in the fibre section, when a patient has diabetes, they are encouraged to eat as many mixed foods as possible, and avoid overeating. Glycemic load is determined by the sheer volume of carbs in a meal as well as the overall composition of a meal. For example, a meal that has only half cup dal and one cup rice will have a higher glycemic load than a meal that has one cup dal, half cup rice, two cups of vegetables and a tablespoon of sesame seed chutney. Now one might say, 'Amita, the second meal literally has more food! How can it be lower in glycemic load?' This is because the portion has now changed to having less rice, more dal (a little more protein), significant quantities of vegetables (fibre!), and sesame seeds (healthy fat). The fibre, protein and healthy fat, combined with the simple carbs in the rice, bring down the glycemic load of the meal.

Ultra-processed foods tend to have a very high glycemic index because they have very little fibre. People often consume such foods in large quantities. For example, when people go out to eat a burger, they usually order fries, a soft drink, and a soft-serve ice cream along with it. So here, one ends up eating a higher volume of food that has a high glycemic index. So, for the fast-food Happy Meal with the soda and ice cream, both the GI and GL are high! And this is also why these foods are harmful to our health, apart from being super high in empty calories!

You've understood the concept of glycemic index and glycemic load, right? Now, let's talk about whether rice is better or roti. We'll use the concepts of GI and GL to understand which one is healthier. Let's take a look!

Food	Glycemic index[8]
Wholewheat atta	50–55
White rice (polished)	70–90

Table 4.2: *Glycemic index*

While the GI of white polished rice is higher than that of wholewheat, we can make it a part of everyday healthy eating by having the rice with lean protein and vegetables. The same applies to roti as well.

Rice

Does eating rice cause weight gain?

The idea that eating rice causes weight gain is a common misconception. Both rice and wheat chapati are sources of carbohydrates. On its own, neither roti nor rice causes weight gain—unless you are eating copious amounts of it, and are loading it with fat. In reality, gaining or losing weight depends on the overall calorie balance—how many calories are consumed versus how many are expended throughout the day.

The rice diet paradox[9]

In the 1940s, Dr Walter Kempner at Duke University treated critically ill kidney patients with a therapeutic diet of white rice, fruit, fruit juices and sugar water—a diet extremely low in sodium and protein.

The unexpected result: Patients lost an average of **141 pounds** despite eating mostly rice and carbohydrates.

The Logical Problem: If rice in particular caused weight gain, then the folks on the rice diet would also have 'gained weight' and not lost weight, right?

This challenges the idea that specific foods like rice inherently make you fat. Weight change depends on overall calories and dietary context, and not individual 'villain' foods.

The real issue with rice is its portion size

No one eats just one or two spoonfuls of rice; typically, a whole bowl of rice is consumed. Eating large portions of rice increases our overall calorie intake.

Additionally, rice is often eaten with pickles, ghee, chips, papads and other accompaniments, which further increase the total calorie count.

A lot of people stop eating 'rice' to lose weight, and some might even come back and tell you that they lost 2–3 kilogramss simply by quitting rice. But the fact is that when they stop eating rice, they are cutting out significant calories as they were not tracking the amount of rice they would take, plus the additional ghee, papad and pickle with it. When people stop eating rice to lose weight, they are actually reducing their total calorie intake, which leads to weight loss.

So, rice is not the culprit; it's the excessive portion sizes and the additional calories from accompaniments that contribute to weight gain.

White rice vs. brown rice: do the same science and concepts apply to both?

The main difference between brown rice and white rice lies in their husk. Just as we eat apples with their skin or without, brown rice contains the husk and the germ, while white rice has these removed. This makes white rice lower in fibre, but gives it a longer shelf life.

Polishing rice increases its shelf life and helps it reach a larger market. However, the fibre difference between brown and white rice is not significant—only about 1 gram. To make up for this difference, you can include extra vegetables or salads in your diet.

Many people believe that eating brown rice helps with weight loss, or is better for diabetes, but in reality, if you consume more calories, you will gain weight and your blood glucose levels will increase, irrespective of whether it is brown or white rice! There is no significant difference between their respective glycemic indices either.

So, if you prefer brown rice, feel free to eat it, but in moderation! Just because it's considered healthier doesn't mean you should eat it in unlimited quantities, as portion control is most important.

Should people with diabetes avoid rice?

Diabetes management is all about keeping blood glucose levels stable.

White rice has a high glycemic index (70–90), which means it digests quickly and causes a rapid spike in blood sugar. Due to the low fibre content, rice behaves like simple starch. Excessive consumption of rice leads to a higher glycemic load, meaning the sugar levels in the blood may rise significantly.

Hence, people with diabetes are advised to consume white rice in limited quantities. Another thing to remember is, if you have white rice, always eat it with lean protein and loads of vegetables. Remember how the fibre in the veggies works on the simple starch in the rice?

What to keep in mind while eating rice if you have diabetes, insulin resistance or pre-diabetes

1. **Portion Control:** Eating rice in smaller portions helps reduce its impact on blood sugar levels.

2. **High-Fibre Options:** Choose brown rice, unpolished rice, or millets instead of white rice to increase fibre intake, which helps keep blood sugar levels under control.
3. **Eat with Protein and Fibre:** Pairing rice with lentils, vegetables or other high-fibre foods lowers its glycemic index, helping maintain stable blood sugar levels.

Leftover rice and resistant starch

This is one Instagram trend that I will back for two reasons: there actually is scientific evidence to support this concept AND it makes the life of the person managing everyone's meals (mostly a woman) easy. There is merit in cooking a large batch of rice, cooling it, storing it in the fridge or freezer, and consuming it in the following days after reheating it. Bring on the egg fried rice, fodnicha bhaat, jeera rice, leftover rice with leftover dal!

What happens to rice when it cools?

In fresh, hot rice, the starch is easily digestible and quickly converts to glucose. However, when rice is cooked, cooled and then reheated, some of the starch converts into 'resistant starch'.

This resistant starch is not easily digestible in the digestive system but is beneficial for the good bacteria in the intestines. As a result, the calories from the rice can be reduced up to 50–60 per cent, and hence its glycemic index is also reduced.[10] A word of caution though, people with diabetes should also understand that whether rice is hot or cold, the main factor that affects blood sugar levels is the quantity of rice (glycemic load) consumed.

The right way to cook rice and its impact on glycemic index

Pressure cooker vs. absorption method

Cooking rice with the 'absorption method' and discarding the starch reduces the starch content. However, only about 2–5 per cent of the starch is removed, so the difference is not significant.

There is no significant difference in the glycemic index between rice cooked in a pressure cooker and using the absorption method.[11]

Does adding vinegar to rice help?

Some people add vinegar to their rice, claiming that it helps slow the blood sugar spike. When food contains acid (such as vinegar or lemon), it slows down digestion a little bit, causing sugar to enter the bloodstream more gradually.[12] This is why the habit of squeezing lemon over dal and rice is beneficial. By the same logic, you can add vinegar to the rice, but remember that adding a teaspoon of vinegar does not mean that your portion of rice can increase. You will still need to portion control the carbs or rice, just that the slower blood glucose spike could be an extra benefit.

Wheat

Does eating wheat lead to weight gain?

The world of Instagram influencers and Whatsapp university will tell you to avoid wheat to lose weight. A lot of you might even have tried it and said, 'Hey, I did indeed lose some weight when I stopped eating wheat.' But this is a very 'deceptive dieting' culture. When people avoid foods made from wheat, they're not just avoiding wholewheat roti or chapati, but also items made from maida (refined flour), such as biscuits, bread, snacks, pizza and pasta. What happens when these foods are eliminated? Consider:

1. The overall caloric intake (total calories) decreases.
2. Foods that are high in calories but low in nutritional value are automatically removed from the diet.

3. Alternatives like rice, jowar, bajra, etc., are included instead.

So, the real issue is not wheat itself, but the control of overall calorie intake! If you eat wheat in moderation, and ensure you maintain a balance of calories and nutrients, weight loss can definitely be achieved. Therefore, the statement that eating wheat leads to weight gain is incorrect. As per my clinical practice, I never tell people to stop eating wheat or gluten to lose weight. In fact, randomly eliminating wheat without truly having any underlying clinical condition can lead to increased gluten sensitivity in the future.

Can you eat wheat if you have diabetes?

Yes, but in moderation! If a person with diabetes eats a lot of maida (refined flour), bread or biscuits, blood sugar levels are likely to rise. However, if you eat homemade roti in moderation, and keep the rest of your diet balanced, there is no problem.

What are celiac disease and irritable bowel syndrome (IBS)

Celiac Disease: Celiac disease is a condition in which the body cannot tolerate gluten—a protein found in wheat, barley and rye. When a person with celiac disease eats foods containing gluten, their immune system reacts and damages the lining of the small intestine. Because of this, the body cannot absorb nutrients properly, no matter how healthy the food is.

Common signs include bloating, loose motions, weight loss, tiredness and anemia.

Irritable Bowel Syndrome (IBS): IBS is a common gut problem where the intestine becomes extra sensitive. There is no damage to the intestine, but it doesn't work normally.

People with IBS often complain of stomach pain, gas, bloating, constipation or diarrhoea.

The symptoms may come and go, and often get worse with stress, irregular eating habits or certain foods.

IBS is not caused by gluten or any allergy. It can be managed with the right diet, regular meals, exercise and stress control.

The key point is that if you are able to digest wheat well without it giving you any allergic reactions, there is no reason to avoid it. But if you find it difficult to digest (like in cases of celiac disease or irritable bowel syndrome), then, of course, wheat should be avoided.

So, wheat is not inherently bad, weight-gaining, or blood-sugar-raising! It's all about how much and in what context you eat it.

Is it true that emmer wheat is lighter on digestion and does not raise blood sugar?

Emmer wheat is a native variety of Indian wheat, and it has a slightly lower gluten content compared to other wheat varieties. This is why some people find it easier to digest. However, assuming that 'lighter digestion' means it doesn't raise blood sugar is a misconception.

Some claim that consuming emmer wheat improves insulin sensitivity or lowers blood sugar. But in reality, there is no solid scientific evidence supporting such claims.

When a person with diabetes starts consuming emmer wheat, they don't just change the wheat; their entire diet and lifestyle changes because now they are trying to eat healthy. They may start eating more vegetables, reduce processed foods, exercise regularly, and lower their consumption of oils like ghee and butter. These overall lifestyle changes are what help control blood sugar, not just switching to emmer wheat.

So, the improvement in blood sugar levels is due to a holistic change in habits, not because of wheat alone!

Should you buy packaged flour from the market, or is freshly ground flour better for health?

It ultimately depends on your convenience and preference. Here's the thing: if you are making roti or phulka at home, whether you use packaged flour or freshly ground flour, the difference in nutritional value is minimal.

What really matters is what you're eating overall. If you're consuming roti but also eating a lot of processed foods like bread, pasta and noodles—which are typically made from refined flour (maida) that offers little nutritional value—it can be harmful to your health. Or ghar ki roti with a restaurant-ordered curry loaded with ghee, butter or cream is not going to turn into a 'health food' simply because it is being eaten with 'ghar ki wholewheat roti'.

As for the concern about preservatives or additives in packaged flour, as long as you're buying FSSAI-certified flour, there shouldn't be any additional harmful substances. Packaged flour may sometimes be coarser, but this doesn't make much of a difference to most people.

If possible, freshly ground flour is always a better option. However, if time or convenience is an issue, there's no harm in using packaged flour. Just ensure to check the expiry date and inspect the flour for any signs of spoilage when opened.

Some households, particularly in places like Gujarat, have mini mills where they grind their own flour. I grew up in Gujarat, and we also had a mini flour mill at home. Aai used to mill all flours at home. If you have the luxury to do so, go ahead. Most mere mortals like me (now) do not have that kind of kitchen real estate, so we stick to our freshly-milled-but-ordered-from-an-online-app kind of situation!

Millets

Sorghum, pearl millet, finger millet, barnyard millet, kodo millet and amaranth are called **millets**. These are considered 'ancient grains' and are gluten-free. With the rise of gluten sensitivity in recent years, there is an increasing recommendation to reduce wheat consumption and incorporate millets into the diet. We also find millets being recommended for people with diabetes due to the notion that wheat causes diabetes. While wheat itself isn't a direct cause of diabetes, processed foods made from it, like bakery items, pizza and pasta, do contribute to health issues. Millets are rich in **fibre**, which helps in improving digestion and controlling blood sugar levels. Therefore, many people are opting for grains like **jowar, bajra** and **nachni** instead of wheat.

Millets contain the same amount of carbohydrates and calories as wheat or rice, but they have higher levels of fibre, minerals such as calcium, iron and magnesium, and B-complex vitamins. Increasing variety in your diet is key to better health, which is why in India, we have a tradition of changing grains according to the season. For instance, ragi or jowar is often consumed in summer, while bajra is the preferred option in winter.

Incorporating millets into your diet not only brings variety but also adds numerous health benefits due to their nutrient-rich profile.

Should you completely stop eating wheat and only eat millets?

Suddenly stopping the consumption of wheat and switching to a millet-based diet can be a bit drastic, as the body is not used to consuming large amounts of fibre, which may lead to digestive issues. In our clinic, we often see people who suddenly stop eating wheat and start consuming high quantities of millets like jowar, bajra and such others every day, and then complain about indigestion, heaviness, constipation, headaches and nutrient deficiencies due to excessive fibre.

Therefore, when incorporating millets into your diet, it should be done gradually and in controlled amounts. Start by consuming millets once a week and then gradually increase the frequency. Sudden inclusion of millets in all meals should be avoided.

So yes, millets are a good healthy choice as they will keep you full for longer due to the higher amount of fibre in them, and they also add variety in terms of taste and nutrient profile, *but* the important thing to remember is not to overdo them. Also, there is a notion that eating millet rotis in place of wheat rotis will make you lose weight by default. This is incorrect. As we have already mentioned, the caloric value of millets is similar to wheat.[13] So, just eating millets is not going to automatically put you in a calorie deficit, nor is it going to work as a magic weight loss pill!

Sorry to burst your bubble, but if you eat too many millet rotis, you will *gain* weight then as well!

What should be the portion size of phulka-bhakri? Is it okay to eat different millets throughout the day?

Similar to what I suggest for wheat rotis, take one phulka, and if you feel more hungry, take another one, but also take more protein in your meal. The same applies to millets like jowar, bajra and nachni.

> Rotis should be about the size of your palm, which is roughly the same size as a regular phulka. If the roti is larger, take half of it, and if it's very large, take a quarter of it.

One important thing to remember: when you are eating wheat and rice as a part of your diet and suddenly start including millets due to health reasons or for variety, make sure to drink enough water. This is because when you start eating jowar, bajra or nachni in the morning and evening, the fibre content in your diet increases, which can lead to constipation. If not managed properly, it can cause issues like fissures. Therefore, remember to drink plenty of water.

Are the various millet biscuits, millet pancake mixes, and other millet products available in the market good for you?

Yes, you can eat millet noodles, pasta, bread, pancake mixes and other similar products. But keep in mind, eating these won't make you a superhero, instantly boost your energy, or provide an exceptionally high amount of protein.

The protein content in both wheat and millets is almost the same. So, eating millets doesn't necessarily give you superior nutrition. However, incorporating variety into your diet is definitely beneficial.

The same goes for children. For ages 1–3, they are typically given wheat and rice, and suddenly shifting their entire diet to millets can cause constipation in some children. This applies to adults as well; any changes to your diet should be made gradually.

Bread or Pav

I'm writing a separate section on bread because in our hectic life, bread is a convenience and is consumed in almost every household. It is often packed for children's tiffins, and there are many different varieties available, but there are also many misconceptions about bread. When I say bread,

I am not talking about Indian breads (roti, phulka, bhakri, puri, chapati, paratha, etc.) but the Western yeast bread loaf. While making fresh phulka or roti for every meal would be ideal, we need to be realistic about the effort and time that go into it, and the fact that we all lead very busy lives, and there is nothing wrong in opting for a little convenience.

Why has commercial or store-bought bread become such a staple in the Indian household? As women have got busier managing work and the home front, the time spent on cooking in the family is steadily decreasing. This is because unfortunately, the primary nutrition responsibilities for everyone continue to be borne by women. Lack of time, skill and ability lead us to the convenience called bread—which is perfectly fine, provided we understand what goes into making bread, and how to make the right choice.

Should bread be eaten every day? Is bread healthy?

The answer to this question cannot be a simple 'yes' or 'no' because it depends on how much and what type of bread you're eating. There are various types of bread available in the market, such as white bread, brown bread, multigrain, sourdough, protein bread, and so on. In the past, many people consumed only white bread or pav, but now there is a greater demand for wheat bread and other varieties.

No matter which type of bread you consume, portion size is crucial. Bread is primarily a source of carbohydrates, which provide energy to the body. Some brown bread in the market contains added colouring, so it may not be entirely made of wholewheat. Even multigrain bread, while a better choice, is still a source of carbohydrates.

Generally, bread contains ingredients like refined flour (maida), water, sugar, salt and yeast. However, commercial bread often contains preservatives, emulsifiers, dough conditioners, gluten and other additives, which can be harmful to health. If you consume four to five slices of bread every day, it can be detrimental to your health. But if you only have a slice of bread or a piece of sourdough bread with an omelette, it is not harmful. Any type of bread, even a healthier variety, should be consumed in moderation.

'Eating in moderation' means not too much, not too little—just the right amount.

It's about balance, not restriction. You don't have to completely avoid your favourite foods, but you also shouldn't overeat them.

For example:

- Having one piece of chocolate is fine, but finishing the whole bar isn't moderation.
- Enjoying fried food occasionally, like once a month, is okay; but eating it every day isn't.

In short, moderation means enjoying all kinds of food, but with control and awareness.

It is important to check the content and types of grains in multigrain bread. Often, it contains only around 10 per cent multigrain flour, and the rest is refined wheat flour and bread improvers—that is like calling a plain paratha a pudina paratha by adding one mint leaf to it! Instead of going for a fancy name, look at the ingredients. Even if a bread is not multigrain but is a regular wholewheat variety, it would be healthier than a 10 per cent multigrain bread.

A good multigrain bread should contain at least 20–25 per cent mixed grains, and the remaining flour should be wholewheat only. While some amount of wheat or refined flour (maida) may be present, if the proportion is appropriate (not more than 15 per cent), it can still be acceptable. It all comes down to reading the ingredients and nutrient label, and understanding how that product is made.

Avoid excessive consumption of bread, especially for people with diabetes or high blood pressure. Remember, more bread means higher glycemic load. Commercial bread often contains high sodium, which can also be harmful for patients of hypertension.

Whether it's bread or roti, portion control is key. One or two slices per day are sufficient; overeating can disrupt the balance of your diet.

When baking bread at home, avoid using gluten or other additives like bread improvers. If you are baking bread at home, you might as well make it from all real food ingredients. Real bread is made using only wheat, salt, yeast and a small amount of sugar. If you are baking it at home, that is all that you should be using.

Does white maida bread stick to our gut?

White bread made from refined flour does not stick to the intestines, but due to the lack of fibre, it becomes 'empty calories'. Therefore, for people with diabetes or those aiming to lose weight, it is better to avoid bread.

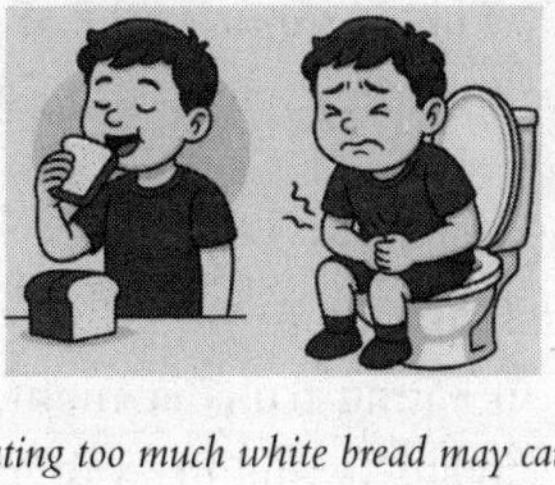

Image 4.4: *Eating too much white bread may cause constipation*

White bread, because it is poor in fibre, when consumed in large quantities (more than 2 slices per day) can cause constipation, especially in young children. The same can also happen with a 10 per cent multigrain, or a bread which is just brown in colour but is actually refined white bread. What used to be older people's problem is now occurring in very young children due to the excessive consumption of empty calories and barely any fibre, in the form of jam or chocolate spread sandwiches. Yes, they are easy to put together—but our children are paying the price for our convenience.

Fruits

We primarily get three nutrients from fruits: natural sugar (fructose), fibre and vitamins. The peel of the fruit contains more fibre than the fruit itself, so whenever possible, one should try to eat fruits with the peel. Of course, this does not apply to fruits like pineapple, but even watermelon rind can be consumed or cooked with, and we should optimise this. We have already seen that it is not easy to meet our fibre requirements, hence when presented with an apple, never eat it peeled!

Is there a 'best' fruit? No. All fruits are great and everyone should aim to eat at least two fruits a day. Research has shown that those who eat fruits are always healthier than those who don't![14] The current world of social media will lead you to believe that there are rules to be followed when eating fruits. Let's explore fact vs. fiction.

Is it okay to eat fruits at night?

There's no harm in eating fruits at night, and no, they do not ferment and create toxins in your gut. In fact, there cannot be a better dessert than a whole fruit (I am not talking about fruit juices). It is going to provide a sweet finish to your meal and also prevent you from digging into the fridge looking for something sweet.

What if you have diabetes? Can you still eat fruit at night? Yes, you can. That's because the meal that you had is now going to act as a buffer and keep your blood glucose levels steady. But this does not mean that you can be gorging on fruits and cream, sugar or ice cream late at night. A small fruit is okay—fruit with extra saturated fat and sugar is not.

Hungry at 5 p.m.? A fruit with some nuts is a better option than a samosa or vada pav. If you don't like to eat fruit as is, pair it with a tablespoon of almond butter, peanut butter, or a cup of yogurt.

Potatoes are not a vegetable but a starchy tuber

'I am not a vegetable'

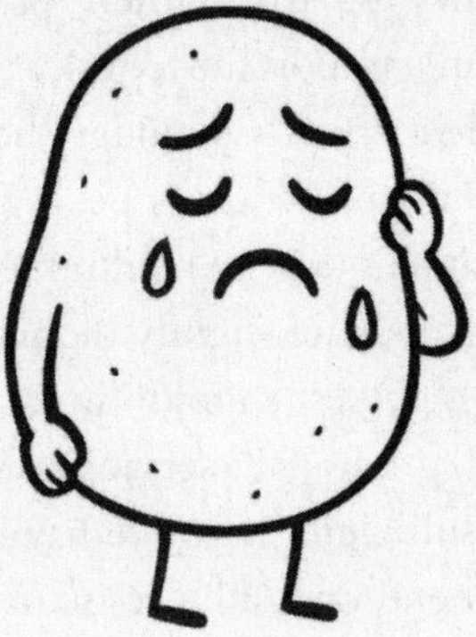

Image 4.5: *Potato as a carb*

In nutrition, potatoes are classified as carbs. If you're eating one potato and one roti, it's like eating two rotis in terms of carb content. And remember, any excess carb in your body that is more than what is needed gets converted into fat and stored. So, it's important to keep track of your carb intake, especially if you're managing your weight or blood sugar levels. That doesn't mean I am calling for a ban on potatoes, but since we are talking of balance, it is important to understand that potatoes with another carb are going to skew the balance of our plate in favour of carbs.

Baked or boiled potatoes with grilled chicken or tofu and vegetables is one of my favourite ways of eating potato. But do note that this favourite meal of mine does not have any other major carb source.

Does eating fruits increase blood sugar? Can people with diabetes eat sweet fruits?

Blood sugar spikes are an important concern, especially for people with diabetes. For individuals without diabetes or insulin resistance, there's no need to worry much, as blood glucose levels naturally rise a little after eating.

When it comes to fruits, their glycemic index and glycemic load are important considerations for people with diabetes. Most fruits fall under the 'low to medium' glycemic index category, such as pears (low GI), mangoes, papayas and pineapples (low to medium GI). However, fruits like chikoo and grapes are slightly higher on the GI scale.

People with diabetes should limit their fruit intake, meaning 200–300 grams (2–3 servings) of a 'low to medium' GI fruit a day is sufficient. If you're having fruits as a snack and you have diabetes or insulin resistance, it's better to pair the fruit with a source of protein or healthy fats, like peanut butter, almond butter, almonds, peanuts or pistachios. This helps reduce blood sugar spikes.

When should fruits be eaten? Can two types of fruits be eaten together? What about milkshakes?

There is a lot of confusion and questions about when to eat fruits and whether it's okay to mix different types of fruits together. Here's the breakdown!

Fruits and their sugar content:

Fruits naturally contain sugar, but it is not the same as the refined white sugar we often worry about. The sugar in fruits is fructose, and it's bound with fibre. This means it's slowly released into the bloodstream, which prevents a rapid spike in blood sugar. So, the sugar in fruits is not harmful in the same way as processed sugars.

When to eat fruits:

You can eat fruits at any time of the day. However, if you have diabetes, it's better to eat fruits after a meal or along with other food. This helps prevent any significant spikes in blood sugar, as proteins and fats in the meal slow down the absorption of sugar from the fruit.

Can two different types of fruits be eaten together?

Yes, it's perfectly fine to mix two types of fruits. Many people enjoy combining fruits like apples and pears, bananas and berries, or even mangoes with pomegranates. There's no harm in combining them, and it can offer a variety of nutrients.

Fruit milkshakes and lassi:

If you enjoy fruit milkshakes or lassi, they can be an addition to your diet as long as they suit your digestion and fit within your overall calorie and sugar intake. For example, a banana milkshake can be a great option as bananas are low in fat and provide a good source of potassium. Just be mindful of the ingredients you add (like sugar or syrups), as they can quickly increase the calorie content. Some people are lactose intolerant, and end up drinking a fruit milkshake or lassi and get indigestion or loosies. In such cases, it is not the mixing of fruit and dairy that is causing the trouble, it is the milk or yogurt by itself which folks with lactose intolerance may find difficult to digest.

Biscuits: Do we really need to eat them?

Biscuits are unfortunately a very common snack. As a nation, we are obsessed with 'fresh food in the morning and evening', but we don't think twice before eating two-month-old (stale) biscuits, that too first thing in the morning. Here's why it's important to rethink their regular consumption.

Excessive consumption and habit:

The biggest problem with biscuits is that it is habit-forming, especially with tea. It's almost a cultural ritual to pair tea with biscuits, and many people consume them mindlessly. The problem intensifies when someone suffering from acidity believes that eating biscuits with tea will reduce their discomfort. In reality, both tea and biscuits—especially with their hydrogenated vegetable oils—can worsen acidity by further irritating the stomach lining.

Biscuits and diabetes: For people with diabetes, biscuits should be completely avoided. There is no biscuit that can truly be considered safe for someone that needs to manage their blood glucose levels. Companies market biscuits with labels like 'sugar-free', 'wheatgrass', or 'ragi' to attract health-conscious consumers, but these still have hidden sugars and fats that can be harmful. Even if they claim to be healthier options, they may not be ideal for individuals with diabetes.

Late-afternoon snacking:
Many people develop a habit of reaching for a few biscuits around 4 or 5 p.m. when hunger strikes. But instead of mindlessly grabbing biscuits, it's better to plan for healthy snacks in advance. When we know we will be hungry around that time, why not prepare or stock nutritious snacks ahead of time? It's always better to plan before hunger hits instead of trying to solve the problem at the last minute. For instance, bringing homemade snacks like roasted nuts, fruits or vegetable sticks can serve as better alternatives to biscuits.

While biscuits may be convenient, they are not the best choice for your health, especially if consumed in excess or regularly.

Can we give biscuits to young children?

Biscuits, particularly cream-filled ones, are a common snack in children's lunchboxes. However, they are not the healthiest choice for kids.

The problem with cream biscuits

Many parents unknowingly pack cream biscuits, puffs or wafer biscuits in their children's snackboxes. These biscuits might seem harmless, but they are far from healthy. Cream biscuits often contain more than 50 per cent fat, most of which comes from hydrogenated vegetable oils, not real cream. This type of fat can have harmful effects on the body, especially for young children whose nutritional needs are still developing.

Savoury biscuits, which some parents think are a better alternative, aren't much better either. They may not contain as much sugar, but are still high in unhealthy fats and salt, which can contribute to issues like obesity, high blood pressure, and poor heart health in the long run.

The role of parents in forming healthy habits

Parents often say, 'Our child doesn't listen; they always demand biscuits.' However, it's important to reflect on how these habits were formed in the first place. Did we teach them to eat biscuits regularly? If you, as a parent, stop the habit of having biscuits as a snack, your child will gradually stop asking for them. It's about leading by example, and making healthier choices at home.

If a child is used to eating biscuits, it's not their fault, it's the pattern that has been taught to them. To break this cycle, change the routine by offering healthier alternatives like fruits, nuts, homemade snacks, or even wholegrain crackers. By gradually replacing unhealthy snacks with better options, children can develop healthier eating habits over time.

In conclusion, while it's convenient to give biscuits to kids, they are not ideal for their health. It's important for parents to educate themselves and their children about healthy eating, and replace processed snacks with more nourishing choices.

Are biscuits healthy?

No, absolutely not! No biscuit is truly healthy, no matter how it's made—whether with jaggery, honey or even clarified butter. Even if you add healthier ingredients like jowar, bajra or protein to the dough, it doesn't make the biscuit healthy. Here's why:

Even if a biscuit or cookie is made at home using millet, ragi, ghee or jaggery, it still remains a product high in refined ingredients. Usually, these recipes call for around 50–70 per cent flour, 15–35 per cent fat, and 10–25 per cent sugar. Whether you bake them yourself or grab them from a so-called 'healthy' brand, they still add extra fat and sugar to your diet—essentially empty calories that our bodies don't really need. This goes for both adults and kids. So, if your child occasionally asks for a biscuit or cookie, feel free to offer a homemade or millet-based one, but keep it in moderation. It's crucial to remember that biscuits, cookies or rusks, no matter how wholesome they claim to be, shouldn't become a daily snack. They should stay an occasional treat, not a dietary habit.

And even biscuits marketed as 'healthy', like those with ragi (finger millet), or digestive biscuits, are not truly good for health. While they may claim to be 'high fibre' or 'sugar-free', they still have fats (usually unhealthy ones) and simple carbs, which can lead to weight gain, poor digestion and other health issues if consumed regularly.

The problem with 'healthier' biscuits

Commercially, biscuits that are low in sugar tend to have higher fat content, and those with low fat generally contain more sugar. This is just basic math behind processed foods. Even if a biscuit tastes bland, it often contains fat or sugar to enhance the flavour. Biscuits are meant to be crunchy and tasty, but they don't provide any nutritional benefits. It only provides us with empty calories. Yes, even the multigrain biscuits.

Even though a roti from yesterday might seem 'stale' and less appetising, it's much healthier than a biscuit that stays 'edible' for months in its packaging. The fact that biscuits can stay 'edible' for months, while freshly made foods can't, is a big red flag about their nutritional value and the additives they contain.

Biscuits, whether made at home or bought from the store, simply don't have any health benefits. It's better to avoid them altogether, especially if you're trying to maintain a healthy lifestyle or if you have conditions like diabetes. It's always better to opt for whole foods like fruits, vegetables or nuts, which provide real nutrition.

Sabudana (tapioca pearls) and its nutrition

Sabudana is a highly refined starch. It is made from tapioca starch extracted from a tuber called cassava, which undergoes a lot of processing. First, the root is washed, then crushed to extract starch, and finally, it is formed into super-processed small balls of pure starch. During this process, the fibre and other nutrients from the cassava root are nearly all removed. As a result, we are left with only pure starch, which we call sago, sabudana or tapioca pearls.

Sago is very easy to digest, which makes it a good option for people who are fasting or sick. Since it digests quickly, it provides immediate energy to the body.

However, it is primarily composed of carbohydrates and lacks other essential nutrients. Therefore, when we consume sago, the sugar levels in the blood can rise quickly. It contains barely any fibre or protein, making it nutritionally insufficient.

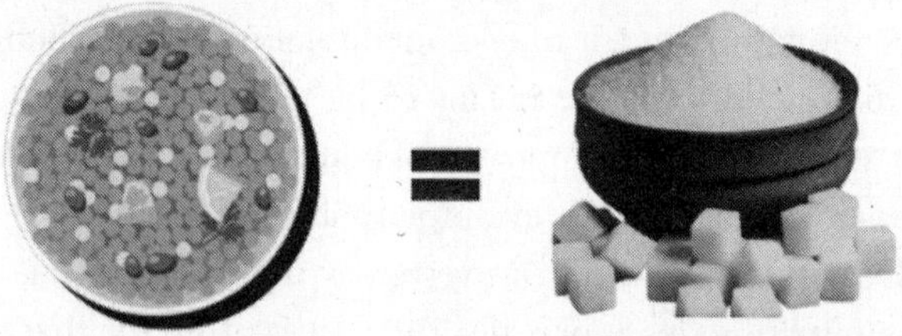

Image 4.6: *Sago as a carb*

Simple Carbohydrates

Is sugar bad and jaggery good?

Sugar and jaggery are essentially the same. Although they taste slightly different, both contain nearly the same amount of calories and have similar nutritional profiles.

Sweetener	Calories (kcal/100 g)	Carbohydrates (g/100g)
White (refined) sugar[15]	**~375 kcal**	≈100 g
Jaggery[16]	**~354 kcal**	≈84 g

Table 4.3: *Comparison between white sugar and jaggery*

Is sugar toxic? What are the side effects of consuming too much sugar?

Sugar is not toxic. However, excessive consumption of sugar increases the risk of various health issues. For example, high sugar intake can create an environment that supports infections because sugar nourishes bacteria and fungal growth.This can lead to problems like urinary tract infections (UTI), fungal infections, and conditions like irritable bowel syndrome (IBS). People who frequently experience such infections should reduce their sugar intake.[17]

Overconsumption of sugar can also lead to skin-related issues. Reducing sugar may help in conditions like dandruff or skin infections. Excess sugar can worsen fungal infections on the skin, and cause other skin problems.[18] Cutting down on sugar can provide relief from these issues.

If your daily intake of sugar or jaggery exceeds 50 grams (10 teaspoons), your total daily calorie intake increases, which can lead to fat accumulation and unwanted weight gain. This, in turn, increases the risk of lifestyle-related diseases.

Can we suffer from a sugar deficiency? Or are there any side effects if we don't eat sugar at all?

There is no direct need for added sugar in the body. Our body does not require sugary foods to obtain glucose. It can derive glucose from complex carbohydrates—especially from grains like rice, wheat, millets and oats. So, there's no need to consume extra sugar. In fact, excess sugar intake only contributes to weight gain and other health problems.

Jaggery contains iron, right?

People have started putting jaggery in their morning chai thinking it will 'boost iron levels'.

Let's be clear: **this is not how iron deficiency is fixed.**

Yes, IFCT says **100 grams of jaggery has 4.63 milligrams iron** and **100 grams of spinach has 2.95 milligrams.**[19]

But nobody, absolutely nobody is eating **100 grams of jaggery**.

That's basically eating a big lump of sugar.

Jaggery is still **sugar**.

No fibre, no meaningful nutrients, just calories.

Spinach, on the other hand, gives you iron **with** vitamins, minerals and fibre—an actual nutrient package your body can use. So, replacing sugar with jaggery, and thinking 'I'm doing something for my iron' is wishful thinking. If iron is your goal, jaggery is not the solution. Spinach and other real iron-rich foods are.

Now we've seen what complex and simple carbohydrates are, their effects and side effects, and why they're needed in our daily diet. We also saw that there's no need to consume more than 2 teaspoons or 10 grams of sugar or jaggery per day. In fact even those two teaspoons are not needed, but I am saying this from experience as a nutritionist that if you allow yourself to have 2 teaspoons sugar or jaggery a day, you will not start obsessing over sweet foods. Having said that, this is a general guideline and not a rule.

We still haven't discussed 'recommended quantities' or 'portion' of food. How much complex carbohydrate should each person eat daily? How much protein? We'll understand that in the next section: ***the Ideal Plate.***

But before that, let's revisit the example of the vada pav diet we discussed earlier. Can you now identify which components in that meal contain carbohydrates?

5

What Should We Cook Today?

The hard truth about adult life is deciding what to eat for breakfast, lunch and dinner, all 365 days of the year. No one can escape it. Even if someone else is cooking—say, you are at a party or a wedding, or you are ordering in—you have to decide what you will choose or how much you will eat. And most of us are trying to eat healthy most of the time, or so I am going to assume, or else you would not have been reading a book on nutrition!

Another fact is that all of us literally eat the same food everyday: a (big or small) portion of protein, some fibre (hopefully!), (healthy?) fats and (complex) carbs. These are the macronutrients that we all eat. If your diet is more on the unhealthy side, you will be eating more added sugars, fats and processed starches, but the basics remain the same. And yet we all also think that we eat very different food every day or at least like to—foodies, you know!

Here's what all this same-same-but-different food does: it keeps some people super healthy, while the majority end up with lifestyle disorders and illnesses. The difference between the healthy and the unwell lies in the proportions of these four macronutrients on your plate. That's what really decides whether your food will protect your health or put it at risk.

And yes, in my book (literally and figuratively), fibre is also a macronutrient.

Some of you who are more aware might be wondering why I haven't mentioned micronutrients yet. That's because if you eat smart, you can ensure that you are getting all your micronutrients—that's your vitamins and minerals as well—while you manage the macros!

What are macronutrients?

Macronutrients are the nutrients our body needs in large amounts. They are the ones that give us energy to work, move and stay active. There are four main types of macronutrients:

Protein: Helps build and repair the body (examples: eggs, meat, tofu)

Carbohydrates: Provide quick energy (examples: rice, roti, potatoes)

Fats: Give long-lasting energy and help absorb certain vitamins (examples: oil, ghee)

Fibre: Keeps our gut healthy and digestion smooth (examples: vegetables, fruits, pulses)

What are micronutrients?

Micronutrients are the nutrients our body needs in smaller amounts. But don't let the word 'micro' fool you, for they're just as important. Think of it like this. To run a car, you need petrol (macronutrients), but without engine oil (micronutrients), the car won't run smoothly.

The two main types of micronutrients are:

Vitamins: Needed for various chemical reactions in the body (examples: vitamin C, vitamin D)

Minerals: Essential for bones, blood and body structure. (examples: iron, calcium)

The Ideal Plate

This is how your main meals—that is your breakfast, lunch and dinner—should look like. You can see that 25 per cent of your ideal plate should be filled with protein, 50 per cent with vegetables, and the remaining 25 per cent with whole carbs.

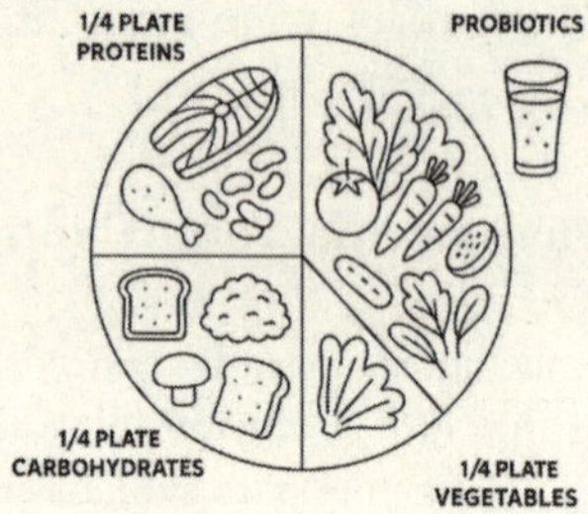

Image 5.1: *The ideal plate*

Balance Your Plate Like This

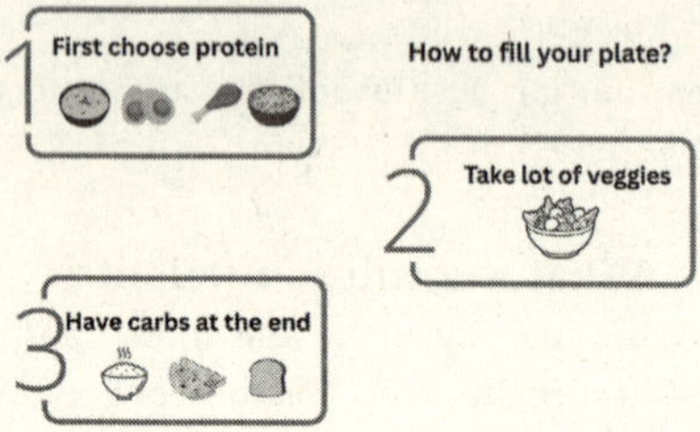

25 per cent protein: Dal, pulses, soybeans, paneer, chicken, fish, mutton.

50 per cent vegetables: This should be the biggest portion on your plate—almost half. And not just one sabzi, include a variety of colours and types.

25 per cent carbs: Rice, roti, bhakri or any other grain.

Now, two groups usually raise their eyebrows here:

1. Protein-conscious folks: 'Only 25 per cent protein? Is that enough?'
2. Roti-sabzi dabba people: 'Do I really need to pack this much protein in every meal?'

Here's the thing: the minimum protein requirement is 0.8 gram per kilogram of body weight. If you actually fill 25 per cent of your plate with protein at each meal (breakfast, lunch, dinner), you'll be well on your way to meeting your needs.

Sample 1

Breakfast: Masala omelette made with 2 eggs
Lunch: 1 bowl of thick moong curry
Dinner: 100 g grilled chicken

Sample 2

Breakfast: 2 besan chillas
Lunch: 1 bowl of thick dal
Dinner: Paneer pulao (with 100 g paneer)

Both the above examples will give you around 40–50 grams of protein. And this is not all that you are going to eat. You will be having more yogurt, some whole carbs and some snack at 4 p.m. So this still offers more opportunities to add protein.

For example, if your weight is 60 kilos, then at 0.8 gram per kilogram of body weight, you need about 48 grams of protein per day. But with the above meals, you're already getting around 45 grams of protein.

So how do you make up for the deficit? Simple!

- At lunch, add 1 cup of homemade curd.
- Around 4 p.m., have a protein-rich snack, for example, 100 g of high-protein yogurt plus 6 or 7 almonds.

This will add another 15–20 grams of protein, taking your daily protein intake to around 60–70 grams.

When you look at fitness influencer videos on social media, it feels like everyone must take whey or protein powders. But if your exercise or physical activity isn't very high, then 0.8 gram per kilogram of body weight is enough. You just need to make sure every meal includes some protein—that's it.

Half Your Plate Should Be Vegetables!

Morning, noon, and night, vegetables need to be on your plate. If you're eating poha or daliya for breakfast, add vegetables. At lunch, include sabzi and salad. At dinner, go for a veggie-loaded pulao with an extra helping of sabzi, salad or soup.

But why this obsession with vegetables? Because research clearly shows that if you want long-term health, your diet must be largely plant-based.[1] In one of my recent podcasts, I mentioned that each of us needs 500 grams of vegetables per person per day. Many people reacted with 'We only buy that much when guests come home!', 'So many veggies will cause indigestion', 'How can we afford it? Prices are so high!' and so on.

Five hundred grams of vegetables per person per day means using 1 cup of veggies with poha or daliya, 1 cup of cooked or sauteed vegetables, and 1 cup of salad at both lunch and dinner.

That already adds up to 500 grams! (And yes, onion and tomato count too.) Now, if you say you can't afford so many vegetables or can't eat that much, I have just one counter-question: can you afford the cost of medicines? Because without vegetables, problems like constipation, acidity, reflux, skin breakouts, acne, dull skin, lacklustre hair and low iron levels are all going to become a part of your everyday life. And then, you will end up spending a bucketload of money trying to fix these issues. And I am not even counting long-term problems like pre-diabetes, PCOS, and high cholesterol that would be waiting right around the corner.

Today in India, even 12-to-13-year-olds are being diagnosed with pre-diabetes. And just like in the US, cases of colon cancer are rising rapidly here too. The good news? A vegetable-rich diet can lower that risk.[2]

Sample 1

Breakfast: Masala omelette made with 2 eggs
Lunch: 1 bowl thick moong curry + 1 bowl sabzi (vegetable dish) + 1 bowl salad
Dinner: 100 g grilled chicken + 2 bowls soup

Sample 2

Breakfast: 2 besan chillas (savoury pancakes) with vegetables
Lunch: 1 bowl thick dal + 1 bowl cucumber curd salad + 1 bowl sabzi
Dinner: Paneer pulao (with 100 g paneer) + 2 bowls soup or 2 bowls raita

Earlier, these menus only highlighted the protein sources. Now, vegetables have also been added.

Why should 50 per cent of your diet be vegetables? Because:

1. **Improves digestion and relieves constipation:** Fibre is essential for gut health.
2. **Covers micronutrient gaps:** Vegetables provide essential vitamins and minerals that reduce the need for supplements.
3. **Boosts plant points:** Vegetables are rich in fibre, earning you valuable *plant points* for better long-term health.
4. **Increases satiety:** High-fibre foods digest slowly, helping control hunger and prevent overeating.
5. **Supports hydration:** Vegetables have a high water content, keeping the body hydrated.
6. **Strengthens immunity:** Fibre feeds good gut bacteria, improving your immune system.
7. **Nourishes skin and hair:** Antioxidants and vitamins in vegetables keep skin glowing and hair healthy.
8. **Protects against diabetes and colon cancer:** Vegetable fibre and antioxidants lower the risk of type 2 diabetes and colon cancer.

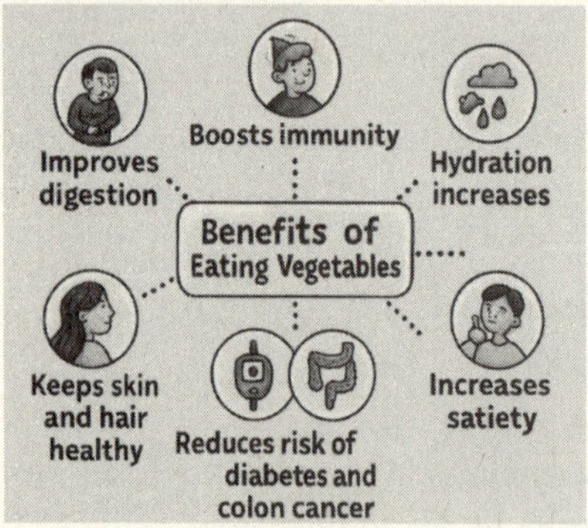

Image 5.2: *Benefits of eating vegetables*

Bottomline, **eat** (don't drink) plenty of vegetables—there is only an upside to it and an absolutely non-existent downside!

Thirty unique plant points

Plant points mean adding more variety of vegetables, fruits, grains, legumes, nuts and seeds to your diet. And everything counts, even the spices and seasonings!

Why is variety important?
It's not enough to just eat tomatoes and cucumbers every day. We need different colours and types of plant-based foods to get a wide range of nutrients. Try to eat at least 30 different plant-based foods in a week.

Why thirty?
The concept is that ensuring a variety of plant-based compounds in our diet plays a crucial role in ensuring that the good gut bacteria in our gut thrive. An average of 30 plant points a week may ensure that we end up consuming different polyphenols, flavonoids, carotenoids, phytoestrogens, phytates, oxalates, etc., all of which are plant compounds essential for the overall health of our gut and, in effect, body.

How to count plant points?
Each unique fruit, vegetable, grain, nut, seed or spice = 1 point

- Fruits: apple, banana, orange, guava
- Vegetables: carrot, spinach, broccoli, beetroot
- Legumes: lentils, beans, chickpeas
- Grains: brown rice, oats, quinoa
- Nuts and Seeds: almonds, walnuts, chia seeds
- Spices: cumin, mustard, black pepper

At the end of the week, aim to score 30 points.

Benefits

- Encourages you to eat a wide variety of foods
- Improves gut health
- Boosts immunity, digestion and overall well-being

In short, plant points are a fun and easy way to diversify your meals and stay healthy![3]

Carbs Should Be the *Last* Thing to Be Added to Your Plate

Yes, carbs should be added at the very end. Why? Because while the main sources of carbs are roti, rice or bhakri, we also get carbs from dals and pulses. The mistake most of us make is this: we fill our plate first with rice or roti, then just add a little sabzi and a little dal on the side. And that's where the balance goes wrong. If carbs fill your plate and stomach first, there's hardly any space left for protein and vegetables. As a result, most people unintentionally eat excess carb calories. This was also proven by a recent study by ICMR, which said that Indians eat too many carbohydrates and their diet is severely lacking in protein and fibre.[4]

Now, you may ask, 'Amita, do we need to count calories while eating home-cooked roti-sabzi?' While calorie-counting has a place for high-level athletes or bodybuilders, the average working Indian does not want or need to get on the six-pack-abs bandwagon. We simply want to be healthy for as long as possible. And hence the answer to everyday calorie-counting is a **maybe**. Food tracking is a useful tool as most of us do not realise the calories hidden in the food we eat, and we do not weigh all that we eat or add. For instance, a dollop of ghee added to dal-rice can mean anything between 1 teaspoon and 2 tablespoons. A dollop is not a standard measure. But my aim here is to make you aware of what is lacking on our plate. We often see that it is easier to focus on what needs to be 'added' than 'removed' or 'avoided'. When it comes to our plate and tummies, the moment we add more vegetables and proteins, we are automatically reducing the space or capacity for other empty calories. So, food tracking or maintaining a food diary is good—weighing and obsessive calorie tracking not so much.

Having said that, we do need to know which food is bringing which majority nutrient to our plate so that we can make an informed choice. If I am trying to reduce my cholesterol and keep topping my breakfast poha with homemade bhujiya without realising that my homemade bhujiya is also deep-fried and packs a punch of oil or fat, I will never be able to achieve my goal. I am telling you to prioritise lean proteins and vegetables in your meals because that's what any dietitian or nutritionist will tell you if they are sane and are practising scientific-evidence-based advice!

The point here is not about eating less of certain foods, but about deciding to eat more protein and vegetables first. When you prioritise them, you naturally end up eating just the right amount of food—not too much. Eating carbs as the last priority does not mean you have to avoid carbs. It only means that you should give priority to protein and vegetables.

The other day, a gentleman at my clinic asked, 'So does this mean I can eat only one roti now?' And I told him, 'No. If you want another roti, that's fine, you can take it. But along with it, you must also take extra dal or chicken (not just curry or gravy), and some more sabzi. Think of it as a "buy 1 get 2 free" offer!'

Sample 1

- Breakfast: Masala omelette made with 2 eggs + 1 phulka
- Lunch: 1 bowl sprouted green gram usal or curry + 1 bowl sabzi + 1 bowl salad + 1–2 rotis
- Dinner: 100 g grilled chicken + 2 bowls soup + 1 bowl rice

Sample 2

- Breakfast: 2 besan chillas with vegetables
- Lunch: 1 bowl thick dal + 1 bowl cucumber raita + 1 bowl sabzi + 1 bhakri
- Dinner: 2 bowls paneer pulao (with 100 g paneer) + 2 bowls soup or raita

What to Do If You Still Feel Hungry?

1. First, check: did you really eat enough protein and vegetables as planned?
2. If you want another roti, add dal and sabzi too. Ask yourself: do I really have the appetite for all that?
3. If you're almost full but still feel like nibbling, start with half a roti, but also add some more sabzi and protein along with it.
4. And as our elders always said, it's better to eat two fewer bites than overeating. The Japanese call it 'hara hachi bu'—eating till one is 80 per cent full.

What About Oils, Ghee and Fats?

As we've already discussed in the fats section, many foods naturally contain some fat. For example, dairy products, non-vegetarian foods (meat, eggs, fish), nuts and seeds like peanuts, almonds, and sesame. When you eat these foods as protein sources, you're automatically getting some fat too. On top of that, we add oil or ghee while making sabzis, pulao, curries, dals, usal, and even rotis. So, there's no need to add an extra fat portion to your plate separately. Remember this thumb rule: oil + ghee (combined) = a maximum of 5–7 teaspoons per day. We don't need more than that.

You might ask: but Amita, how can we manage cooking like this every day?

The real key to a healthy diet is meal planning. Think of it like school canteens: they always put up a weekly menu. Similarly, if we plan ahead, it's half the battle won. And you don't even need to plan for the entire week in one go. Start with just three days. That way the planning won't get overwhelming and you will also have time or gaps in case there is any sudden change of plans, any food left over or such.

The biggest benefit of meal planning is that you do not have to wake up to a gigantic existential question like 'What should I cook or eat today?' Instead, you will wake up to 'Today's lunch is chicken and dinner is tofu!' This also helps if you have kids in the family. Everyone in the family already knows what's coming for lunch or dinner. It brings discipline and structure to eating habits. Without meal planning, what happens especially with kids is that they keep demanding something new every day. Like my son says, 'If I ate dal-sabzi-roti for lunch, can I please have something different for dinner?' So, to avoid that daily headache, plan your meals in advance.

How to Do Meal Planning

1. First check what's at home: work with what you already have.
2. Think of family needs: elders may need softer, lighter meals; kids might need energy-rich ones.
3. Balance nutrition: make sure proteins, vegetables and fibre are included in every plan.

If you don't plan, you end up having to make three food decisions every day (breakfast, lunch, and dinner). But if you plan ahead, you make that decision once every 3 days, and life gets easier.

One simple hack: divide your week into 3-day blocks. Make a meal plan for each block.

That way, you spend less time deciding and more time enjoying healthy, balanced meals.

How to Plan Meals (Menu Planning) with Nutrients in Mind?

The first thing to fix is your protein source. Where are you getting protein from? It could be from dairy products like paneer or curd, from pulses and lentils, or from non-vegetarian foods like eggs, chicken, and fish. Soy-based options are also available. Let's say you are planning meals for the next 3 days, Monday to Wednesday. For every meal, first finalise the protein.

For the last 10–15 years, my breakfast has been 2 eggs along with 1 chapati. If chapati isn't available, I take a slice of toasted bread (no butter). Why? Because the protein from the eggs is essential for me. Once protein is decided, plan which vegetables will go with it. After protein and veggies are in place, decide whether you want rice, roti, or bread along with it. Most of us do the opposite: we first decide whether we want rice or roti. But the right approach is to start with protein, then add vegetables, and finally choose carbohydrates.

By planning meals this way, every meal will be balanced and complete. You can be sure that you're meeting all your nutrient requirements in every single meal.

SAMPLE MENU

Monday		
Breakfast	**Lunch**	**Dinner**
2 Egg Omelette + 1 Slice of Sourdough toast OR 2 Besan Cheela + Green Chutney	1 Cup Dal + 2 Cups Stir fried veggies + 1 Roti	100 g Grilled Fish / 1 cup Spicy Soy chunks + 1 Cup Soup + 1/2 cup cooked Quinoa
Tuesday		
Breakfast	**Lunch**	**Dinner**
1 cup Overnight Oats	1 Cup Sprouts + 2 Cups Diced veggie salad + 1 Thepla	100 g Tandoori Grilled Chicken / Grilled Paneer + 1,5 Cup Rice Pulao (Add 1 cup diced veg-gies)

Why Do Colours Matter When Planning Meals?

When I see photos of people's meals, most of the time everything is the same colour. And that's not ideal. If you're planning your meals, try to include different colors on your plate. For example, if you're making cauliflower today, which is usually yellowish because of the turmeric added to it, don't pair it with yellow lentils. Choose whole masoor instead. Also add a beet or spinach salad—now you've added another color. Even a slightly tart vegetable like green amaranth can add variety. The idea is that when you take a photo of your plate, there should be at least three different colours. Why? Different colours don't just make your plate look good; they give you a range of polyphenols and other beneficial nutrients that are great for your health. Plus, the way the food looks also forms a large part of its palatability and appeal—we do want our food to look appealing every day!

Your fridge and freezer are your best friends

There's a common myth that food stored in the fridge or freezer goes stale or loses its nutrients. That's completely wrong! Fridges were invented to keep food fresh for longer, not to destroy its nutrition. Frozen or refrigerated foods do not lose nutrients just by being in the cold storage.[5] In fact, fruits and vegetables, if left out, tend to spoil quickly; that's when they lose nutrients—not in the fridge! Some water-soluble vitamins like vitamin C may reduce slightly during freezing or cooking, but here's an easy fix: squeeze a little lemon on cooked vegetables before eating. In today's busy lives, getting timely and balanced meals is tough. That's why the fridge and freezer are your best friends!

How to Meal Prep

1. Store vegetables smartly:
   Wash, chop, and store in airtight containers in the fridge.
   Some vegetables, like peas or beans, can go into the freezer for longer storage.
2. Cook and store lentils and pulses:
   Cook, cool, and freeze.
   Reheat when needed.

3. Prepare sauces and pastes:
   Chutneys and pastes (like ginger-garlic) can be made in advance and stored in the fridge.
   Use them directly while cooking meals.
4. Store cooked meals:
   Cool leftover meals and store in airtight containers in the fridge.
   Reheat and eat the next day.
   Freezers can store them for longer periods.
5. Prepare fruits:
   Wash, cut and store in the fridge.
   Ready-to-eat fruits are perfect for a quick snack.

The fridge and freezer save time, help you eat balanced meals, and reduce stress. Meal prep is a simple way to take care of your health while staying on schedule!

'But Amita, you still haven't told us anything about micronutrients like vitamins and minerals! I have a B12 deficiency, and my doctor has suggested injections. How can I get it from my diet?'

Let's see, this is where micro support systems come into play!

6

(Not So) Micro Support Systems

When we speak of health, there are macronutrients, micronutrients and supporting factors which impact our holistic health. Supporting factors like our environment, sleep, stress, pollution, the water we drink, our mental health, access to services—are all important determinants of our health.[1]

If you look at the ideal plate we discussed earlier, it doesn't spell out exactly *how much* of each micronutrient (vitamin or mineral) you need. Why? Because if you eat according to that plate every day, you'll automatically cover most of your vitamin and mineral needs, except maybe two vitamins and two minerals.

But what exactly are these micronutrients—vitamins and minerals—and why do we need them?

Consider micronutrients as electricity in your home. You don't notice how many devices are running at the same time using electricity until there's a power cut. Suddenly, you realise that life comes to a standstill without electricity. Vitamins and minerals work the same way in our body. As long as you get enough from your diet, everything hums along smoothly. But when levels drop, even the tiniest processes in your body start slowing down.

Vitamins are like the essential workers in your body; they are part of almost every process happening inside you. Minerals? They form the structure as well as the tools for the efficient functioning of your body. Both are absolutely essential for your body to run like a well-oiled machine.

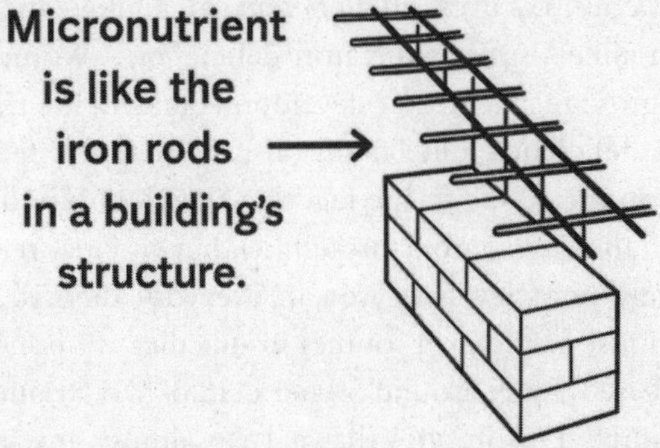

Image 6.1: *Micronutrients are like the iron rods in a building's structure*

Minerals like sodium and potassium are so essential that if our body runs out of them, we simply cannot survive. If iron levels drop too low, even breathing becomes a struggle. Low calcium makes our bones weak and affects our heart's ability to function properly. And if magnesium is lacking, our muscles feel constantly tired, and even simple daily movements leave us exhausted.

Essentially, minerals are like the currency of our body: just as our world cannot function without money, our body cannot function without these essential elements.

The good news? Most minerals are available in sufficient amounts in our daily diet. In fact, compared to protein, carbs and fat, our body needs minerals in much smaller quantities, which is why we group them under micronutrients.

Common Mineral Deficiencies

1. Iron
2. Calcium

Iron

In our country, over 50 per cent of adults—men and women alike—suffer from iron deficiency.[2] Women and young girls are at a greater developmental and life risk due to iron deficiency. One might assume that women have poor iron levels due to the fact that they lose blood every month (and hence iron through it), but the real reason is extremely poor levels of iron in everyday diet. To top it all off, most of the iron sources in our diet are non-heme (plant-based), only around 50 per cent of which our body can absorb.[3] This implies that it is an almost unwinnable situation where women and their iron levels are concerned, and one of the biggest factors is that women are largely vegetarian, or even if they're non-vegetarian, they barely eat a significant quantity of animal-based food due to various socio-economic reasons. To top it all off, exercise levels are extremely low in women, leading to very poor muscle mass and hence poor levels of muscular iron storage in the body.

The fact that every woman is constantly trying to get slimmer adds fuel to the fire called iron deficiency because the first thing that gets sacrificed in the pursuit of remaining skinny is FOOD! Constant dieting and low food intake also leads young women and girls to have irregular periods, scanty and painful periods, and significant pains associated with premenstrual syndrome. Low iron also leads to low hemoglobin, and you may notice symptoms like fatigue, lack of focus, dizziness, hair fall, pale or dull skin, or even brittle nails. In young children and young adults alike, poor iron levels also lead to lower IQ and mental performance.[4]

Iron deficiency anemia isn't just a women's issue; kids and men can also be affected, mainly due to insufficient iron in their diet.

Recommended daily intake of iron:[5]

Men: 19 mg/day

Women: 29 mg/day

There are two types of dietary iron:

- **Heme iron**: Found in animal-based foods, easily absorbed by the body.
- **Non-heme iron**: Found in plant-based foods, not absorbed as efficiently.

Since many of us eat mostly vegetarian diets, and those who eat eggs or meat do so in very small amounts, iron deficiency has become extremely common.

Solutions:

- Take iron supplements or tablets if needed.
- Increase iron-rich foods in your diet (see sources of iron listed below).
- Avoid drinking tea or coffee with meals, as they can reduce iron absorption.[6]
- Pair iron with vitamin C to boost absorption.[7]
- Iron supplements should be taken with a bit of lemon juice for better iron utilisation.

Sources of iron

Animal-Based (Heme Iron):

- Liver: especially chicken or goat liver
- Red meat: beef, mutton
- Chicken
- Fish: especially sardines, tuna, mackerel
- Egg yolk

Plant-Based (Non-Heme Iron):

- Nuts: almonds, pistachios, cashews
- Seeds: flaxseeds, pumpkin seeds, sunflower seeds
- Figs, black raisins
- Lentils and legumes
- Leafy greens: spinach, amaranth (rajgira), fenugreek leaves, radish greens

Calcium

Calcium is the mineral that builds strength in our body. It keeps our bones, teeth and muscles strong, and ensures our nerves and heart work smoothly. It's also the unsung hero behind blood clotting, energy production, and hormone regulation.

We get calcium from a variety of foods:

- **Grains:** ragi, sorghum (jowar), pearl millet (bajra), wholewheat
- **Seeds:** sesame, pumpkin seeds, melon seeds
- **Nuts:** almonds, walnuts, pistachios
- **Dairy and eggs**

Fun fact: Milk isn't necessarily the *highest* source of calcium; grains and seeds often give more!

Ragi gives you **364 milligrams**. Amaranth leaves give **330–72 milligrams**. **Til seeds** hit **1,283 milligrams**. **Niger seeds** reach **572 milligrams**. Now compare that to the usual favourites: buffalo milk has **121 milligrams,** and paneer has **476 milligrams.**[8]

So, if you're chasing calcium and only relying on milk, you're playing on the wrong team. The real calcium leaders are sitting in your kitchen in the form of grains and seeds.

For vegetarians or those who are lactose intolerant, millet, seeds and fortified foods are excellent options.

Recommended daily intake of calcium:[9]

- Adults: 1,000 mg/day
- Children: 500–550 mg/day (depending on age)

Signs of deficiency: Brittle nails, hair fall, white spots on nails, and general weakness. Always check your calcium levels before starting supplements.

Supplement tips:

- Calcium citrate is safer than calcium di-phosphate (lower risk of kidney stones).[10]
- Calcium acetate is also a quick absorption option.
- **Caution:** Too much calcium can cause kidney stones.[11] Always consult a clinical nutritionist before taking supplements.

Remember, bone health isn't just about calcium. Vitamin K2, zinc, magnesium, phosphorus and regular strength training all play a role.[12]

Vitamin B12 Deficiency

This is what a patient was saying at my clinic the other day: 'Even if you go to the doctor for a cold or cough these days, they often end up prescribing B12 tablets. It seems like there is a B12 deficiency epidemic going on.' It might seem like a new 'fad' or 'trend' in medicine, but the reason B12 deficiency was not so common or widely spoken about earlier is because there simply wasn't enough data. It is only in the past two decades that we have realised the important role that vitamin B12 plays in our energy management, and how its deficiency can actually make us feel super weak. Studies have shown that 75 per cent of people in India have B12 deficiency.[13]

This isn't a new fad, it's new information. As medical research has progressed, we have understood how crucial B12 is for our health. Tests for B12 are now widely available, and many people do have a deficiency.

B12 is key for managing our body's energy cycles and immunity. If it's low, you might feel weak, tired, and forgetful, lack focus, or experience tingling in your hands and feet.

Recommended daily intake of B12:[14]

Men and women: 2.2 mcg/day

Vitamin B12 sources:

- **Non-vegetarian foods:** Chicken, fish, eggs, milk and dairy products
- **Supplements:** B12 can also be obtained from nutritional yeast or other synthetic supplements. Many vegans have this notion that B12 supplements are made from animal sources, but they are not. They

are synthetically derived compounds made in a lab. So, if you have a B12 deficiency, the best thing to do is to take a supplement.

So, how do you know if your body is B12 deficient? Don't assume deficiency just because your diet is low in B12. Your body *can* produce some B12 naturally, but some people cannot produce enough of it to meet daily needs. Deficiency usually happens because your intrinsic factor—a protein needed to absorb B12—is low.

For B12 deficiency, doctors usually prescribe a **1,000 mcg tablet**, and if the deficiency is severe, injections may be given. And no, B12 tablets aren't meant to be taken at night; they can actually interfere with your sleep if you do!

Vitamin D3

Vitamin D3 is naturally produced in our body when we get sunlight. In a country like ours, with an almost year-round availability of sunlight, deficiency shouldn't happen. But it does, and here's why:

- We don't spend enough time outdoors.
- We lack regular exercise.
- Our diet may not provide enough calcium, magnesium or protein to support natural vitamin D synthesis.
- Many of us spend the whole day in air-conditioned offices.

Where do we get vitamin D3 from?

Vitamin D3 comes from dairy and non-vegetarian foods. You can also get a small amount of a precursor called ergocalciferol from almonds, walnuts, seeds, and oils, but honestly, it doesn't do much to boost your D3 levels.

If your D3 is low, you might notice poor sleep, feeling tired or weak all day, low energy in your body's natural cycles and, most important, soft or weak bones. Low D3 can also make blood sugar management harder.[15,16]

Vitamin D3 is available as tablets or liquid supplements. Since vitamin D3 is fat-soluble, always take it with some healthy fat. A daily dose of 1,000 IU or booster dose of 60,000 IU once a week is recommended. If you're not deficient, there's no need to take supplements unnecessarily. One key thing to remember: taking D3 supplements for too long without need can cause toxicity.

Our Supplement Needs

When it comes to supplements, most of us are confused about what we actually need. Walk into any pharmacy and you will see shelves overflowing with bottles promising better health, more energy, stronger immunity and faster recovery. But do we really need all of these? Let's break them down to understand what they are, whether you need them, and how much to take if you do.

Zinc

Zinc is a mineral that your body needs for many important functions. Think of zinc as the handyman of the body. It helps with repair work like immunity, wound healing, skin health, and hair growth—even taste and smell depend on it.

Do I recommend it?

Most Indian adults need around 13.2–17 milligrams of zinc per day.[17] A cup of cooked rajma contains about 2.5

milligrams of zinc, but your body might only absorb half of that due to the phytates. Animal sources like chicken or fish provide better zinc absorption, but these are not consumed daily in most Indian households.

My recommendation: for most healthy individuals, food sources are enough. But in case of frequent colds, hair fall linked to low zinc, or confirmed deficiency, a short-term supplement under clinical guidance may help. Too much zinc can actually reduce copper levels and harm immunity, so this is not a 'more is better' supplement.

Selenium

Selenium is another trace mineral—meaning your body only needs small amounts of it. It helps make important proteins that protect your cells from damage and support your thyroid function (the gland that controls your metabolism).

Do I recommend it? No.

The requirement is tiny, around 40 mcg per day.[18] And here's the interesting part: you can meet this need from just 1–2 Brazil nuts a day. Eggs, fish, whole grains and dairy also contain selenium.

Food sources are usually enough. Supplements only make sense when there is a diagnosed deficiency or specific thyroid-related indications under medical supervision.

B-Complex

B vitamins are like the spark plugs of your energy system. They help your body convert food into usable energy and support nerves, skin and red blood cells.

You will find B vitamins in:

- milk and curd
- eggs
- meat and fish
- whole grains
- dals and legumes
- nuts and seeds

If someone is constantly tired, often gets mouth ulcers, or follows a very restricted diet (which I do not recommend unless medically required), a B-complex supplement can help.

Do I recommend it?

In many Indian diets, especially vegetarian ones, B12 intake is low. So, a B12 supplement may be useful after testing, particularly for those who don't eat meat or dairy regularly. But again, it should not be taken blindly. And opting for B12 is not the same as randomly taking a B-complex supplement. Remember: your priority should always be improving food quality.

Multivitamins

A multivitamin looks like an easy solution: 'I'll just take one pill and cover everything.'

But here's what really happens: if your diet is already decent, that multivitamin usually adds nothing extra. It just gives you very expensive urine. Most vitamins in these tablets are present in such small amounts or forms that your body doesn't absorb them well.

On the other hand, if someone eats:

- very little fruits and vegetables,
- minimal protein,

- mostly packaged food,
- or follows fad diets

The multivitamin gives them a sense of security but doesn't fix the root problem—the food itself.

Do I recommend multivitamins? Almost never.

Instead of spending money on a tablet, improving meals gives far better results. Supplements cannot provide fibre, phytonutrients, protein quality, or healthy fats that real food offers. A multivitamin may help in certain situations, like recovery from an illness or in case the diet intake is very low due to medical reasons, but it should not be a long-term habit.

L-Carnitine

L-carnitine has become extremely popular in urban India, especially in gyms and fitness centres. Walk into any supplement store and you will find multiple brands of L-carnitine promising rapid fat loss. But does it actually work?

Your body naturally produces adequate L-carnitine, and you also get it from foods—particularly chicken, mutton, fish and dairy. Vegetarians have lower L-carnitine levels than non-vegetarians, but the body compensates by producing more on its own and conserving it better. There is no evidence that vegetarians suffer any health problems from lower L-carnitine levels. The marketing claims around L-carnitine are far stronger than the scientific evidence backing it.

Let's be clear. L-carnitine helps transport fat to cells to be used for energy. But this process only works efficiently when:

- you are eating enough protein
- you are exercising regularly, especially strength training

Without these, L-carnitine does nothing noticeable.

Do I recommend L-carnitine for fat loss? Not really.

For the vast majority of Indians, L-carnitine supplements are not necessary. Save your money. Whether you are vegetarian or non-vegetarian, your body is producing adequate amounts. For athletes, it would be a different story, depending on their training and diet.

Berberine

Berberine is often marketed as 'natural metformin'. It is a plant compound that helps improve how the body handles glucose and insulin.

What this really means:

- it may help reduce blood sugar spikes
- it may improve insulin resistance
- it may slightly lower cholesterol
- it may support fat loss in people with metabolic issues

Sounds impressive, but here's the catch. For most individuals, fixing meal patterns, increasing protein and fibre intake, and walking after meals gives equal or better results.

Do I recommend it? No.

Apple Cider Vinegar (ACV)

ACV is one of the most overhyped supplements out there. Other than being used in a salad dressing or to clean up a particularly grimy oven, it is pretty useless.

Claims:

- burns fat
- improves digestion
- detoxifies
- boosts metabolism

Reality:

ACV does **not** burn fat. It does **not** detoxify anything—your liver and kidneys already do that. So, what does ACV actually do?

It may help slightly reduce blood sugar spikes when taken before meals, especially before high-carb meals, by slowing digestion. But the effect is mild.[19]

You can get a similar or better result by:

- eating more fibre
- adding lemon to meals
- including protein in every meal
- walking for 10 minutes after eating

Do I recommend ACV?

No, not as a supplement. If someone likes the taste and uses it in cooking or dressings, that's fine. But drinking ACV shots can:

- damage tooth enamel
- irritate the stomach
- worsen acidity

There is no need to force yourself to consume it. ACV is not a weight-loss solution.

Omega-3

Omega-3s are among the few supplements most people can benefit from, especially if their diet lacks fatty fish.

These fatty acids help reduce inflammation, protect the heart, and support brain function. They also improve triglycerides which we see many Indians struggling with.

What do Omega-3s do?

- Reduce inflammation
- Improve heart health
- Lower triglycerides
- Support brain function
- Improve joint stiffness or soreness

Who needs Omega-3 supplementation?

- People with chronically high triglycerides
- Those who rarely eat fish
- People with joint inflammation

Do I recommend it? Yes, if required. Omega-3 is one of the few supplements with strong evidence and very low risk when taken in appropriate doses. Here's the detail most people skip: the EPA:DHA ratio matters. Some research suggests that omega-3 supplements with a higher EPA:DHA ratio reduce certain inflammation markers.[20]

Magnesium

Magnesium is a mineral involved in over 300 enzymatic reactions in your body. It's essential for muscle and nerve function, blood sugar control, blood pressure regulation, and bone health.

Signs you might be low in magnesium

Many people with mild magnesium deficiency don't show dramatic symptoms. But there are a few common patterns you may recognise:

- Trouble falling asleep or waking up tired
- Muscle cramps, especially in calves

- Constipation
- Headaches or migraines
- Feeling 'tired but wired' at night
- PMS mood swings or cramps
- High stress levels
- Eyelid twitching

These don't always mean magnesium deficiency, but magnesium often helps.

Do we recommend it?

Magnesium is one of the few supplements that can genuinely improve day-to-day quality of life, sleep, digestion, stress and muscle comfort. But it should still only be used under supervision. For quite a few people, magnesium supplements do not work.

We recommend magnesium supplementation if:

- Sleep is consistently poor
- Muscle cramps or tension are frequent
- You struggle with stress or anxiety
- Your diet does not include nuts, seeds, and leafy greens daily
- You drink 2–3 cups of tea or coffee a day

For everyone else, food sources are usually enough.

Nutritional Yeast for Vitamin B12

Nutritional yeast has become popular among vegetarians and vegans because it is often marketed as a plant-based source of Vitamin B12. But here's an important detail many people don't know:

- Nutritional yeast naturally does NOT contain B12.
- It only contains B12 if the manufacturer fortifies it.

So, the benefits depend entirely on the brand and whether B12 has been added.

What does nutritional yeast do?:

- It provides a cheesy, umami flavour
- It is a good source of B-vitamins (other than B12)
- It contains protein and fibre
- It works well in vegetarian cooking

Who actually benefits from it?:

- Vegetarians and vegans who do not consume eggs or dairy regularly
- People who want a flavourful way to increase B-vitamins
- Those looking to replace cheese in certain recipes

Do we recommend it for B12? Only if the product is clearly labelled as B12-fortified, and the B12 content per serving is mentioned.

Even then, it may not be enough to correct a deficiency. For Indian vegetarians who already have a high risk of B12 deficiency, direct B12 supplementation is usually much more reliable.

Nutritional yeast can be a good addition to the diet, but it should not replace proper B12 supplementation if levels are low.

Collagen

Collagen is a structural protein: think of it as the 'glue' that holds your skin, joints, hair, nails and tissues together. As we age, natural collagen production decreases.

Your body will make collagen if it has the right building blocks: amino acids (particularly glycine, proline and hydroxyproline), vitamin C, zinc and copper. So, eating a protein-rich diet with adequate vitamin C and minerals might be just as effective as taking collagen supplements. The most important thing to understand is this: **your body doesn't absorb collagen supplements as collagen. It breaks it down into amino acids, then rebuilds what it needs.**

So, collagen supplements can help, but only if protein intake from food is already adequate.

Do I recommend it? Collagen is helpful *only* when the foundations—your protein intake, hydration, sleep, and basic skin care—are already in place. It is not a substitute for eating enough protein. We recommend collagen for joint support and recovery much more than for cosmetic skin benefits, which vary widely.

Moringa Powder

Moringa powder is just dried, powdered drumstick leaves. When you remove the water, nutrients get concentrated, so 1 teaspoon gives you the nutrition of a big handful of fresh leaves.

But here's the part people forget: **moringa powder is not a magical supplement.**

If your goal is better nutrition, you're almost always better off eating the actual vegetable. Fresh leaves give you **fibre, bulk and satiety**, the things a powder can't.

And moringa capsules or tablets?

They're just tiny doses of the same powder. Unless you have a genuine appetite issue, difficulty eating greens, or are following specific medical guidance, they don't serve much practical purpose. They're simply a way to sell what fresh sabzi could have given you anyway.

Safety?

In normal food quantities, moringa is safe. But very high supplemental doses can cause digestive issues, lower blood pressure, or interact with thyroid medications. More is not always better.

Ashwagandha

It's classified as an adaptogen, meaning it's believed to help your body manage stress. In recent years, it has gained significant attention in the wellness world. Ashwagandha has been studied primarily for stress and anxiety reduction, and the results reflect that. It may help lower cortisol levels (your primary stress hormone), reduce anxiety symptoms, improve sleep quality, and potentially support thyroid function. Some studies also suggest benefits for strength and muscle recovery in people who exercise regularly, though the effects are modest.[21,22] However, these studies had smaller sample sizes and varied dosages. Its long-term effects are yet to be studied.

Wheatgrass

Wheatgrass is the young grass of the wheat plant, harvested before it develops grain. It's often juiced and consumed as a shot, or sold as a powder. Walk into any health food store or juice bar, and you'll find wheatgrass being promoted as a detoxifying, energising superfood.

What it does: wheatgrass contains chlorophyll, vitamins (particularly A, C and E), minerals and amino acids. Proponents claim that it detoxifies the body, boosts immunity, aids digestion, and increases energy levels. The reality is far less impressive than what the marketing suggests.

Do I recommend it? No, not as a supplement. There's very limited scientific evidence supporting the dramatic health claims made about wheatgrass. Most of the 'research' consists of small, poorly designed studies or is based purely on its nutrient content rather than actual health outcomes in humans. I strongly discourage everyone from drinking wheatgrass juice as it can potentially increase your risk of kidney stones.

The truth about wheatgrass: yes, it contains nutrients, but nothing you can't get from eating regular vegetables.

While vitamins and minerals are important for our health, there are other factors like good, deep sleep and regular exercise that also play a very important role in maintaining or ruining our health. Let's dive deeper into both of these topics!

Sleep

Impact of sleep on health

Adequate, deep sleep is essential for the body's repair and recovery. Lack of sleep can cause fatigue, irritability and reduced concentration.

Sleep and weight

Inadequate sleep disrupts hormonal balance, increases hunger, and may lead to weight gain. That's why good sleep is vital for weight control.[23]

Sleep, inflammation and cortisol

Poor sleep raises cortisol (the stress hormone), which can increase inflammation.[24] Long term, this can contribute to several health issues.

Sleep and gut health

Lack of sleep disrupts the balance of gut microbes, leading to digestive issues and other health complaints.[25]

Exercise

What's the best exercise?

The best exercise is the one **you enjoy and can stick to regularly.** Yoga, swimming, cycling, running, walking over 5 km, gymming or dancing are great options.

How to choose the right exercise?

Base it on your health condition, preferences and goals. Consult a healthcare provider before starting, especially if you have health concerns like hypertension, dyslipidemia, knee pain, heart conditions, high cholesterol, obesity, diabetes, and so on.

Benefits of Exercise

- improves heart health
- manages blood sugars
- strengthens muscles and bones
- improves sleep
- improves body balance and mobility
- improves gut health and functioning of vital organs
- reduces stress
- enhances overall well-being

How to build muscle?

Eat a protein-rich diet and include strength training (weight lifting). Always do these under proper guidance.

How to reduce fat?

A balanced diet plus cardio exercises (like running or cycling) help reduce excess body fat.

Exercise and blood sugar control

Regular exercise improves insulin sensitivity, helping regulate blood sugar levels.[26]

Strength training and women

Strength training means lifting weights to build muscle strength. For women, it's especially important, as it increases bone density and lowers the risk of osteoporosis.[27]

Water and hydration

The human body is made up of about 60 per cent water. In men, 60–65 per cent of the body is made of water, and in women, around 50–60 per cent (due to higher fat percentage) is made of water. Staying hydrated is essential for energy, metabolism and overall health.

Importance of water for health

Like fuel for a car, water is the fuel for our body. It keeps every system running smoothly.

Energy and cellular function

- Water powers your cells and supports essential chemical processes in the body.

- It regulates body temperature and keeps you cool, especially on hot days.

Water and weight

- Appetite control: drinking enough water helps you feel full and reduces unnecessary snacking.
- Metabolism boost: adequate hydration supports metabolism and helps burn fat more efficiently.[28]

Dehydration, inflammation and cortisol

- Lack of water stresses the body.
- Inflammation: dehydration increases inflammatory responses, leading to swelling and other issues.[29]
- Cortisol: low hydration raises cortisol (the stress hormone), which negatively impacts health.[30]

Water and digestion

- Gut balance: adequate water helps maintain healthy gut bacteria.
- Bowel movement: proper hydration keeps stools soft and ensures smooth digestion.

Best ways to stay hydrated

- Water: aim for at least 2–2.5 litres daily. Check the colour of your urine—it should be clear or very pale yellow.
- Fruits and veggies: cucumbers, watermelon, oranges, apples and other high-water foods.
- Soups and porridges: add hydration and aid digestion.

Role of sodium and ORS

- In hot weather or after exercise, water alone may not be enough—sodium is also needed.

- ORS (oral rehydration solution): a mix of water, sugar, sodium and minerals that restores electrolyte balance and provides quick hydration.
- Sodium's role: it helps maintain fluid balance and supports cell function.

Precautions for hydration

- Choose: water and natural sources like coconut water, buttermilk, etc.
- Avoid: sugary drinks (soda, energy drinks) as they cause weight gain and health problems.

Hydration and its impact

- Hormonal balance: adequate water keeps hormones regulated and lowers stress.
- Skin: well-hydrated skin stays healthy, glowing, and wrinkle-free.
- Hair: hydration adds strength and shine, reducing breakage and hair fall.

What happens if you drink too much water?

Drinking water is essential—but too much of anything can be harmful, and water is no exception!

If you drink more water than your body actually needs, important minerals like sodium get diluted. This can cause weakness, headaches, dizziness and other issues.

Think of it like an overinflated balloon: if you keep adding air, it bursts. Similarly, overloading your body with water puts stress on your cells, and that can be dangerous.

7

The Anti-Inflammatory Diet

Many lifestyle-related disorders that we see globally today, like diabetes, high blood pressure, heart disease, PCOS, hypothyroidism, arthritis, and so on, are all linked to chronic inflammation at their root.

What is inflammation? Imagine a mosquito or bee bites your skin. The area becomes red, swollen and warm. This is your body's response to the 'attack'. This same process is called inflammation.

If this kind of inflammation persists inside the body, in organs or tissues, it can lead to chronic inflammatory disorders. It might start as something simple like an upset stomach or gas and progress to serious conditions like atherosclerosis (heart disease).

Most medications are anti-inflammatory, meaning they help reduce or control inflammation, giving the body a better chance to heal from within.

Diet plays a huge role here. If your diet is mainly anti-inflammatory—rich in whole foods, plant-based ingredients, fresh fruits and vegetables, and healthy natural fats, your body heals faster.

Another major cause of inflammation is a weakened digestive system. When digestion is strong and efficient, the production of harmful substances is minimised. A diet rich in prebiotics and probiotics supports the gut to produce compounds that neutralise toxins and reduce the impact of inflammatory foods.

That's why the digestive system is often called the 'second brain'. When your digestion works well, you feel more satisfied, balanced and happy.

Lifestyle Diseases and the Anti-Inflammatory Diet

These days, obesity, diabetes, high blood pressure, high cholesterol and heart disease are all on the rise. And the main reason? Huge changes in our lifestyle.

In earlier times, people didn't eat so frequently. Meals were usually taken once, twice or at the most three times a day. Food was scarce, poverty was common, and people managed with whatever was available.

Today, the situation has flipped. We have money and choices, and with that, our eating habits have also completely changed. Ultra-processed foods, fast food, and outside meals have become a daily affair.

We've almost stopped eating simple home-cooked meals. Instead, have replaced them with chow mein, biryani, burgers and pizza. Add to that a sedentary lifestyle: earlier people walked or cycled; today, we sit in front of a computer all day long, and don't even manage 2,000 steps in a day. Exercise has become a distant memory.

On top of this, stress levels have skyrocketed—work pressure, poor sleep, binge-watching Netflix at night, endless scrolling through reels and videos. All of this takes a heavy toll on the body.

Of course, lifestyle diseases existed in previous generations too. Diabetes and obesity weren't unheard of. But back then, diagnostic tools weren't easily available. The common 'test' was if ants gathered where someone urinated; people would assume, 'Oh, they probably have diabetes.' Today, we have better diagnostic tools, which is why the numbers look even higher.

Another big issue is obesity. Most people today are either overweight or what we call skinny fat—meaning their weight looks 'normal' but their body has more fat than muscle. Because of this, insulin resistance has shot up, and many people now fall into the prediabetic category.

Where diabetes used to show up at 50–60 years of age, we now see it in 12-to-13-year-old children. The culprits are unhealthy diet, lack of exercise, and an overall imbalanced lifestyle.

All these factors together are driving diabetes rates to alarming levels worldwide. And sadly, our country is right at the top of the charts. About 589 million adults (aged 20–79 years) worldwide are living with diabetes. According to the International Diabetes Federation (IDF) Diabetes Atlas 2025, 11.1 per cent, or 1 in 9 of the adult population (20–79 years), is living with diabetes, with over 4 in 10 unaware that they have the condition.[1] According to the World Health Organization (WHO) India, about 77 million adults in India currently live with diabetes, and nearly 25 million are estimated to have pre-diabetes (high risk).[2]

Why Does Diabetes Happen?

There are two main reasons for diabetes: the body produces too little of the hormone insulin, or insulin is present but the body doesn't use it properly. This is what we call insulin resistance. Both of these lead to the same outcome: diabetes.

There are two main types of diabetes:

1. **Type 1 Diabetes**: In this type, the body cannot produce enough insulin. Because of this, blood sugar cannot stay under control. Insulin is a hormone that plays a very important role: it helps carry glucose (blood sugar) from the bloodstream into the body's cells, where it is used for energy. When insulin is lacking, glucose cannot enter the cells and instead keeps building up in the blood. This rise in blood sugar is what we call diabetes. That's why, when fasting blood sugar or random blood sugar is checked in people with this condition, it is usually found to be high.
2. **Type 2 Diabetes**: This was earlier known as 'adult-onset diabetes' because it usually appears after the age of 40. But now, things have changed. Type 2 diabetes is increasingly being seen at a much younger age, even in teenagers. In most cases, it starts with **insulin resistance**. This means that insulin is present in the body, but it doesn't work properly. The receptors on the cells, which normally recognise and respond to insulin, stop responding well due to various reasons. As a result, glucose cannot move into the cells and keeps accumulating in the blood, leading to rising blood sugar levels. If your fasting blood sugar is above 120 mg/dL, or your post-meal blood sugar is above 140 mg/dL, it indicates the beginning of diabetes or insulin resistance.[3]

Obesity greatly increases insulin resistance.[4] Insulin works like a school teacher. Imagine a noisy classroom: when the children start making a lot of noise, the teacher

Glycated hemoglobin (HbA1c) and fasting insulin

Glycated hemoglobin (HbA1c):
Our blood always has some amount of sugar (glucose) in it. This sugar sticks in small amounts to hemoglobin (the protein in red blood cells that carries oxygen). The sugar-coated hemoglobin is called glycated hemoglobin.

Think of it like making sugar syrup. If you keep it aside for some time, sugar crystals begin to stick and form again. Similarly, if blood sugar remains high for a long time, sugar begins attaching itself to hemoglobin.

So, HbA1c is the measure of sugar 'stuck' to hemoglobin. It reflects the average blood sugar level in the past 3 months.

If your HbA1c is high, it means your blood sugar has been consistently high over that period.

Fasting insulin:
Insulin is an important hormone that carries glucose from the blood into the body's cells, where it can be used as energy. Fasting insulin measures how much insulin your body produces on an empty stomach.

If your fasting blood sugar looks normal (low), but your insulin levels are high, it means your body is working extra hard to keep sugar under control.

This test shows how much insulin your body needs to produce just to maintain fasting sugar levels.

When insulin levels are high, but the body doesn't respond to it properly, this condition is called insulin resistance.

comes in, scolds them, and the children immediately listen and sit quietly. Similarly, after a meal when blood sugar levels rise, the 'teacher' insulin arrives and instructs the glucose to move into the muscles (this process is called glycogenesis). If your blood sugar is normal, then just like children listening after one warning, glucose quickly leaves the blood and enters the muscles when insulin signals it.

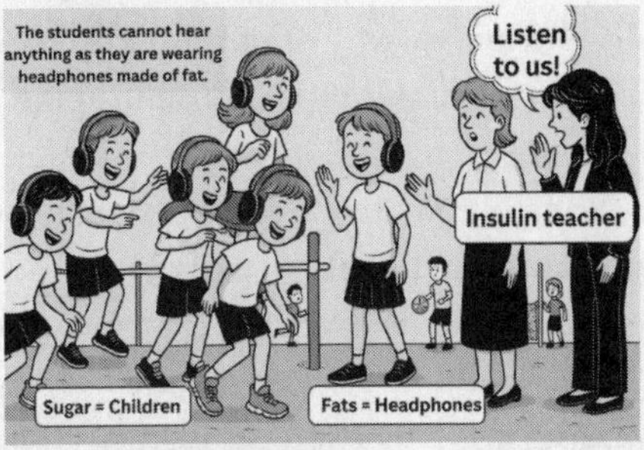
The students cannot hear anything as they are wearing headphones made of fat.
Listen to us!
Insulin teacher
Sugar = Children
Fats = Headphones

Image 7.1: *The blocking effect of fat on insulin signaling*

now imagine the teacher is shouting, but the kids are wearing headphones, so they can't hear a thing. When our body fat increases, it's like putting 'headphones' on the insulin receptors in our body. Insulin's instructions don't get through, and glucose doesn't know where to go. As a result, blood sugar levels stay high, even though insulin is trying to do its job.

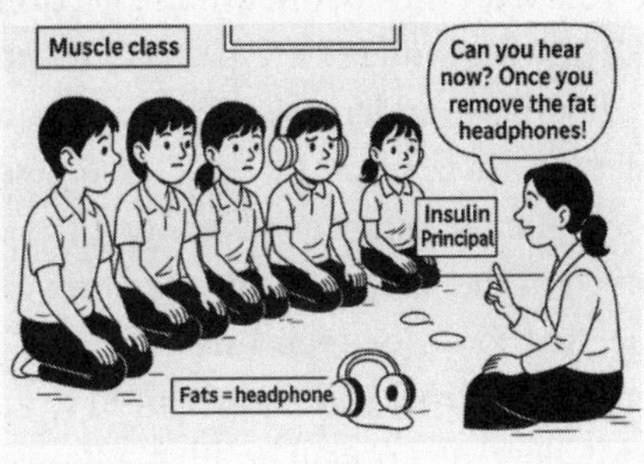
Muscle class
Can you hear now? Once you remove the fat headphones!
Insulin Principal
Fats =headphone

Image 7.2: *How dropping fat helps improve insulin action*

When a person with insulin resistance or diabetes manages their diet and exercise, and reduces body fat, it's like removing the headphones. Glucose can now 'hear' insulin's instructions again. This is called increased insulin sensitivity. It's essentially the body's way of consistently trying to keep glucose levels in check and reduce insulin spikes.

What Do You Need to Do to Keep Your Blood Glucose and Insulin Levels Steady?

You need to eat a diet which is balanced for protein, fibre, healthy fats and carbs, as explained in the previous chapter. You also need to exercise regularly and work on maintaining and preferably gaining muscle mass so that you have more muscle where insulin can send the glucose to. You can also start redeveloping the ancient Indian practice of walking for 15 minutes after a meal. The world and social media might tell you that you need to be monitoring your blood glucose spikes using devices like continuous glucose monitors (CGM), but you really don't need to do that. If you eat the way I have explained, your sugars *will* remain steady. CGM devices are recommended only if you have uncontrolled diabetes and are on insulin injections, and even in those cases, I recommend my patients to stop wearing them once they have understood the positive impact of a balanced diet on their sugar levels. This obsession over a 'normal blood glucose spike' needs to stop.

As explained in the image below, when you eat a diet full of ultra-processed foods or high carbohydrates, your blood sugars shoot up like a rocket. What we need to achieve for a healthy HbA1C level and overall health is a steady merry-go-round after our meals. That can very easily be achieved with a slight modification of the ideal balanced meal plate.

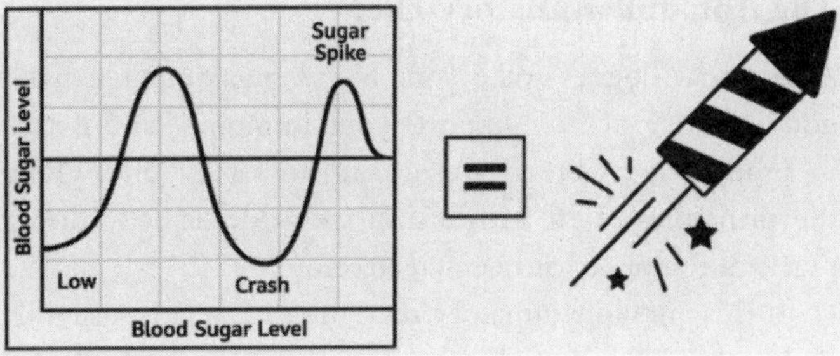

Image 7.3: *Illustration of blood glucose spikes and crashes*

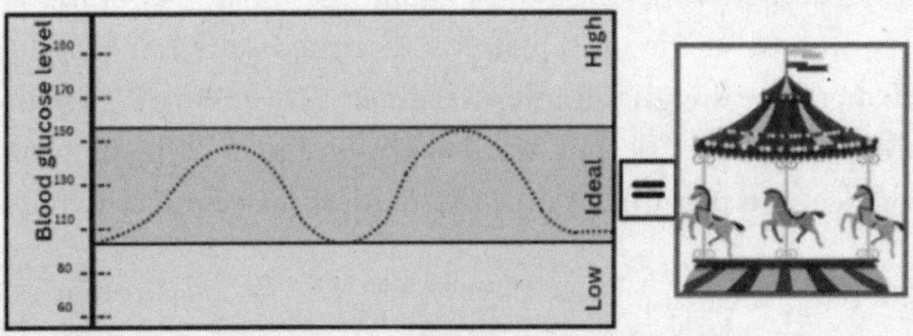

Image 7.4: *Cyclical blood glucose levels*

Diet to manage diabetes: It's obvious that in this diet, we need to cut down on simple sugars or added sugars. Simple carbs like sugar, refined flour, and bakery items are quickly absorbed by the body, causing a rapid spike in blood sugar. But just as quickly, the sugar drops, leaving you tired and craving food again.

On the other hand, complex carbs, like whole grains, lentils and vegetables, along with protein and healthy fats, keep blood sugar levels steady and slow, like riding a merry-go-round at a smooth, pleasant pace. This prevents fatigue, keeps you full for longer, and reduces the urge to snack repeatedly. A balanced diet leaves you feeling more energetic and refreshed throughout the day.

The Anti-Inflammatory Diet

A diet that doesn't spike your blood sugar quickly, has a good balance of fats, supports your immunity, and is rich in protein and fibre is an anti-inflammatory diet. Using the principles of an anti-inflammatory or diabetic diet, a practical template has been created for you.

In this anti-inflammatory diet, protein intake is slightly higher than that in the balanced ideal plate, carbs are lower, fibre is abundant, and oil or fat use is minimal. Actually, this kind of diet works for almost all lifestyle-related conditions. If you look at the ideal plate we discussed earlier, managing diabetes or weight simply means: slightly increase protein, keep vegetables as they were, slightly reduce carbs like roti or rice, and pair this healthy diet with some physical activity.

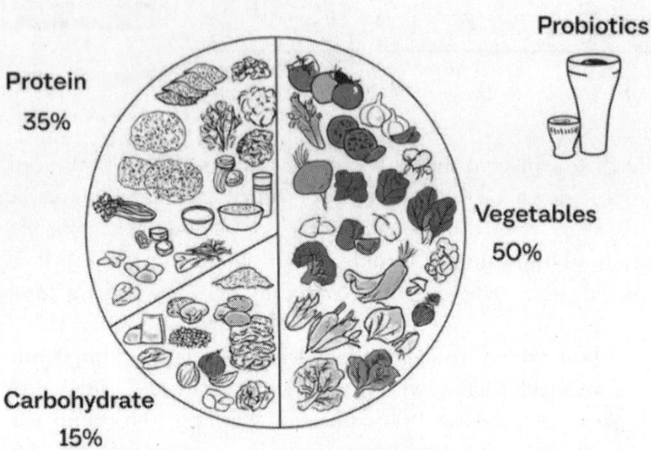

Image 7.5: *Ideal plate*

In all lifestyle-related conditions, our insulin metabolism is often a bit off. So, it's best not to put extra stress on an already weak system with too many carbs. That's why carbs should be slightly reduced. At the same time, increasing protein is very important, because when there's a disease or hormonal imbalance, our organs are under stress and need extra strength. Hence, protein intake should be boosted.

As for vegetables, we've already discussed why they're essential. To support immunity and gut health, it's crucial to get fibre and polyphenols from vegetables. And if you add probiotics like buttermilk or yogurt—well, that's the cherry on top! There's no need for extreme measures like drinking bitter gourd juice or eating just once a day to stay healthy. Small, sensible changes are enough.

8

How to Eat

According to the marathi shloka 'Vadanikavala gheta', which is said before meals, food is not just for filling the stomach ('udarbharan nohe'), but should be consumed like a sacred ritual ('janije yajnakarma'). Just as a yajna (sacred fire ritual) is performed slowly and mindfully with calmness, eating should also be done with care and attention. Food is not just calories, it's the foundation of good health.

Food keeps us alive, gives us the energy to carry out our daily activities, and brings family and friends together. It's part of every important moment in life, whether joyful or sad. For many of us, our love for food drives us to travel, cook, watch food shows, attend cultural events, join food clubs, and more. Unfortunately, these days, food has also become a source of many health issues.

Nutrient supplements are temporary fixes, not permanent solutions.

The world we live in, where Instagram filters make everything look perfect, and instant gratification gives us quick dopamine spikes, real food often doesn't feel like a

'quick fix'. That's because true, wholesome food works slowly. Real change happens gradually.

And honestly, most of us don't have the patience for it: we want to try something, see results immediately, tweak, observe, and repeat. Reading about it alone feels exhausting; we've become so impatient!

We crave instant solutions. It's not entirely our fault that wellness industries constantly promise us **'lose two sizes in 9 weeks', 'reverse diabetes in a month', 'drink this to fix your thyroid', etc.**

But many of us have already felt the downsides of these quick fixes.

What really needs to change is our approach to true, sustainable health. How, what, and how much we eat matters. My approach to food and diet, which has proved effective for thousands of clients worldwide over the years might seem simple, but it truly works.

1. Eat only when you're hungry.
2. Eat slowly, without any distractions.
3. Eat calmly until you feel satisfied.
4. Eat within a limited time.
5. Choose minimally processed, whole and diverse foods.

Eat Only When You're Hungry

Hunger is the most basic need of the human body—even newborns cry when they're hungry.

But as we grow older, the habit of 'eating by the clock' sets in, breakfast at 9, lunch at 1, dinner at 8.

In today's fast-paced lifestyle, where most of our time is spent sitting in front of computers, we eat because it's mealtime, not because we're hungry. And that's where the trouble begins.

Most of us no longer wait until we're actually hungry

I meet many people who say, 'I feel like I'm always hungry', and they feel guilty about it, but in reality, it's guilt about eating constantly.

Hunger and eating are completely natural and healthy processes, so there's no need to feel guilty.

The real problem is that most of us don't truly recognise what 'hunger' is. We eat when we're thirsty (thirst confusion), bored, tired, it's 'mealtime', watching TV, stressed, or driven by emotions.

In truth, you should eat only when you're genuinely hungry

In my nutrition programmes, I ask clients: 'When you feel hungry, what exactly does your body feel? What are the symptoms of hunger?'

Nine out of ten people have no idea.

When you dig a little deeper, answers start to emerge: 'My stomach is rumbling', 'My stomach feels tight or empty', 'I feel a bit dizzy or low on energy', 'I get irritable', 'I can't focus', etc.

But it takes time and reflection to notice these signals.

Then I ask: 'When was the last time you truly felt hungry?'

Most people respond: 'I don't remember.'

When we eat before hunger even strikes, we place a huge nutritional and caloric load on our body, one it hasn't asked for and isn't prepared to digest yet.

It's like pressing the accelerator without changing gears, the car isn't ready to move forward. This sudden load puts enormous stress on our digestive system. And the big boss of this system? Insulin.

Insulin is a powerful boss; it decides where the nutrients in the body should go.

Working under insulin are its little assistants: digestive enzymes. They get clear orders: 'Process this food as quickly as possible.'

Then these digestive enzymes call in bile, acids and other enzymes, and the whole system goes into a full-blown food-processing war mode. And all of this…where does it go?

Into the body's big warehouse—that is, the fat deposits

Boss insulin is always on alert: 'What if no food comes? What if you starve yourself?' So, it stores extra nutrients in the body as fat.

The more excess insulin you have in your body, the more fat gets stored. Fat is the body's only way of storing energy for the long term.

Your body uses proteins, vitamins and minerals for daily needs, and anything extra, whether it's carbohydrates, proteins or fats—gets stored as fat.

> Yes, even excess protein in the body gets stored as **fat**—not as muscle!
>
> To actually build muscles, you need consistent daily exercise; protein alone won't do it.

What happens when you wait until you're really hungry?

When you wait until genuine hunger strikes, you give your body the time to recognise its nutrient needs, prepare for digestion, and decide how to use and distribute nutrients efficiently. At that moment, your body signals the 'hunger cue' and is fully ready.

Because your body is prepared, insulin and its helpers don't react hastily, so digestion flows naturally and smoothly.

No excess digestive juices or insulin are produced, meaning:

- no acidity,
- no insulin spikes,
- no reflux,
- no uncomfortable heaviness,
- less gas or bloating,
- and you don't crave food again within an hour of eating.

Of course, it's not that simple, but this is the first step toward healthy digestion.

When not to eat?

Emotional eating is on the rise. Eating to feel better or to cope with emotions doesn't solve the real problem. We often turn to instant noodles, ice cream or biryani for temporary relief. The biggest consequence of emotional eating is **guilt**:

- 'Did I overindulge?'
- 'I've lost control!'
- 'I must have gained 5 kilos now!'

(You rarely hear anyone say, 'I ate a salad as comfort food!')

We know that emotional eating doesn't solve our problems; in fact, it often adds more negative feelings on top. Yet, almost all of us have given in to emotional eating at some point.

How to deal with it?

Ask yourself: **Am I 'BAH SALT'?**

- **B:** Bored
- **A:** Anxious
- **H:** Hungry
- **S:** Stressed
- **A:** Angry
- **L:** Lonely
- **T:** Tired

If the answer is hungry, then eating is appropriate, but the meal should be nutritious and balanced.

If the answer is anything else, it's better to use non-food strategies instead of eating.

I tell my clients:

When you feel like deviating from your usual healthy eating pattern, ask yourself: Am I anxious? Stressed? Angry? Feeling lonely? Tired?'

If the answer is yes, choose something from your self-care menu first before thinking about food.

Create your own SELF-CARE menu:

- Write in a diary (journalling)
- Tidy up your wallet or purse
- Listen to a favourite song
- Water the plants
- Take a warm shower
- Create a new playlist
- Spend time with pets or children
- Read a book
- Stand on the terrace, balcony or by a window, look at the sky, and take deep breaths of fresh air

There are plenty of options, the point is: **try doing at least one of them first**. And if you still feel like eating, **don't deny yourself**, just eat **mindfully, slowly and consciously**.

There's no more reliable way than this.

Eat slowly and without distractions

If you have a phone and internet or Wi-Fi, this advice is especially for you. We live in a world where answers come instantly, everything is just one click away, and this habit naturally seeps into our meals and overall lifestyle.

Nowadays, even making a simple meal feels like a chore. Cooking has become 'work', and even buying the ingredients feels like a hassle.

I ask my clients: 'When was the last time you had a calm, satisfying, and joyful meal?' Some remember a day or two, but many stay silent because food has now become just a 'fix', a way to distract from problems.

We've forgotten the joy of searching for recipes, taking time to cook leisurely, enjoying the process, and truly savouring our meals. That's one reason the food processing industry grows at 11.18 per cent annually (Annual Survey of Industries, 2018–19), and why non-communicable diseases are rising just as fast in India. It's no surprise.

Eating slowly gives your body the chance to digest food properly and absorb nutrients efficiently. Naturally, not overeating also supports this. Remember: good digestion is the foundation of good health.

So, what does 'eat slowly and without distractions' really mean, and why is it important?

Most of the time, when we eat, our attention is elsewhere—preparing food for family, talking or scrolling on the phone, working or watching TV, etc. Our focus is constantly divided.

Eating mindfully without distractions allows your body to digest food better, absorb nutrients fully, and ultimately support overall health and satisfaction.

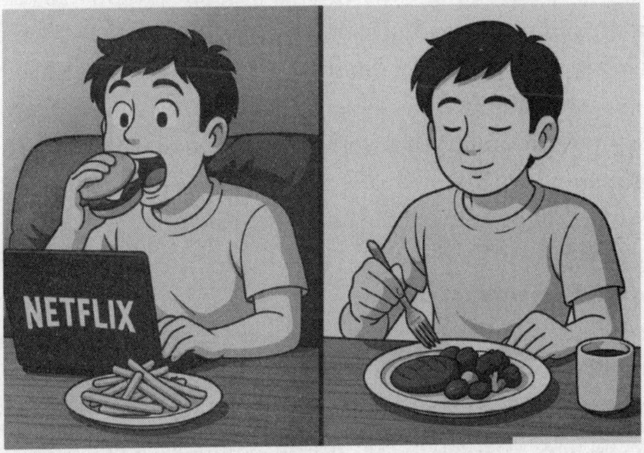

Image 8.1: *Avoiding distractions while eating*

This habit has become so common that it even defines things like a 'Netflix binge'—eating mindlessly while watching something.

But when you eat calmly and without distractions, you are fully present in the act of eating. You enjoy the process even if the food on your plate isn't your absolute favourite, and you eat consciously. Your attention is on your body's natural signals of hunger and fullness. I firmly believe that food is not just about filling the stomach—it nourishes both body and mind.

So, why do you feel like reaching for something sweet or extra right after a 'TV dinner'? Because when you eat while watching your favourite show, your brain doesn't properly register that you've eaten—the 'fullness signal' from your brain gets missed.

At that moment, the sense of satisfaction, joy and satiety that you should have felt doesn't happen.

The act of eating then becomes mindless eating, instead of the intended mindful eating—eating with full awareness. This is why, even after finishing a meal, you immediately crave something sweet or crunchy. And of course, there's also the possibility that your meal did not have adequate protein which also increases the chances of a sweet craving, but lack of mindful eating also has a role to play.

Sounds familiar, right?

Another side effect of eating while watching TV or scrolling on your phone is that we eat much faster. Have you ever noticed that in pubs, the music is always loud, fast-paced, and energetic? The reason is simple: when you are distracted or your brain is 'lost in the music', you eat more and faster. Similarly, when we eat while engrossed in TV or a movie (think: popcorn at the cinema), we tend to eat really quickly without realising it.

Even talking on the phone while eating speeds up your eating because eating and talking at the same time creates a distraction. Seems like common sense, right? Yet many of us do this habitually.

Your brain quickly learns once you start eating while doing something else, the next time you repeat that action, your brain immediately cues: 'It's time to eat.'

For example: at the movies with cheese, butter or caramel popcorn. You don't even realise it, and halfway through the film, you've eaten the equivalent of a full meal! Try a simple experiment: take the same amount of popcorn, sit down without TV or phone distractions, and eat slowly. You'll immediately notice how little you actually need to feel full. You'll think, 'That's enough!'

The same goes for eating ice cream or chips while watching TV. These are learned food cues from your brain.

That's why it's crucial to only focus on eating when you eat. No multitasking, no distractions.

Eat slowly—until you feel satisfied, not stuffed

In one study, it was found that eating fast is associated with higher body weight, poor metabolic markers, and a generally unhealthy diet preference.[1]

Here's a powerful insight: if you eat slowly, and without any distractions, putting down your fork or spoon after each bite and not taking the next bite until the previous one is chewed and swallowed, you can reduce your food intake by about 40 per cent. When we think about losing weight, the first advice is usually 'eat less!' This method is extremely reliable, and all my clients notice the difference from the very first follow-up. They say: 'Since we started eating slowly, we eat much less and now realise how much we used to overeat!' You might think these 'eating rules' are too simple. That's perfect, because simplicity is the key. Nothing more is needed.

Even more important is the rule 'Stop eating when you feel satisfied'. Don't eat till you feel stuffed, like 'I need a deep breath after eating' or 'My head feels like it will fall into the plate'. Growing up, many of us heard 'Don't waste food on your plate'. That's a good habit, but here's a trick: if half a roti or portion is left and you're already satisfied, take only half to begin with. Food isn't going anywhere. This way, you stay in control, you decide how much to eat.

Across cultures, healthy traditions teach the same: don't overeat. In Marathi, the shloka 'वदनी कवळ घेता' teaches it, and Tibetan monks are taught to eat slowly and take two fewer bites than needed. Overeating makes us sluggish. Eating until satisfied keeps the body light, the digestive system happy, and provides proper nutrition and energy. That's the purpose of eating to nourish yourself. An unexpected benefit? You feel happier, cortisol (stress hormone) drops, and your body experiences less strain, because it isn't overloaded with excessive food.

Eating until satisfied naturally helps you practice portion control

If you've ever looked at general advice on weight loss or fitness, you'll often hear the term 'portion control'. Simply put, it means avoiding overeating. But when we eat quickly, distracted or highly processed, very flavourful foods, sticking to a reasonable portion becomes really difficult. Another challenge is that the 'serving size' mentioned on a packet is usually very different from what people actually eat.

For example, a serving of breakfast cereal might be 30 grams (half a cup), but how much we actually pour depends on hunger, habit or sometimes no thought at all. This mismatch is called portion distortion, and the solution is mindful eating.

When you eat slowly, consciously and fully engage all your senses, you naturally feel satisfied, so you can stop before overeating and avoid filling your plate beyond what your body truly needs.

How to eat slowly?

If eating with hands: Don't pick up the next bite until the current one is fully chewed and swallowed. It seems simple, but it really works.

Put down your fork, spoon or knife after each bite: This gives you a short pause to take a sip of water, chew properly and savour the flavors.

Don't mix all food together at once: In India, we often mix dal, vegetables, curd and rice into one big heap. Instead, mix small portions at a time. This helps you eat slowly and stop before overeating.

Eat as if it is a wine tasting: Imagine food tasting is like wine tasting. Just as you don't drink an entire glass at once, do the same with food. Pay attention to the flavour, aroma and different notes of food. This makes you more mindful and slow while eating.

Engage in conversation, eat like the French: If eating with others, chatting naturally slows you down. (But remember: don't talk with food in your mouth!)

Set a timer: Track how long it takes you to finish a meal and consciously slow your pace.

Use a 'pace-setter': Like running in a group behind the slowest runner, match your eating speed to the slowest person at the table, often children!

Use apps if helpful: There are apps that guide you to slow down and track meal duration. Avoid looking at your phone while eating.

Time-restricted eating

Many of us think we eat for about 12 hours a day, but in reality, it's often much longer. For example, if you wake up at 7 a.m., by 7.30 a.m. you might already be drinking tea or coffee. Most people continue eating until at least 10 p.m. During weekends, movie nights or binge-watching sessions, eating can stretch past midnight. A great first step to better eating habits is time-restricted eating—limiting food intake to a set window of about 12 hours. For instance, start at 8 a.m. and finish all your meals of the day by 8 p.m. This 12-hour eating window is also helpful for people working in shifts.

Benefits of time-restricted eating:

- Improves metabolism
- Helps digestion (avoiding eating right before sleep)
- Enhances sleep quality
- Keeps you light and energetic through the day
- Reduces acidity, bloating and gas
- Diminishes dark circles and puffy eyes
- Keeps you active and enthusiastic
- Helps regulate hormones more effectively
- Makes medicines work more efficiently if you're on them
- Balances your circadian rhythm (natural body clock)
- Promotes a calmer, more satisfied and happier state of mind

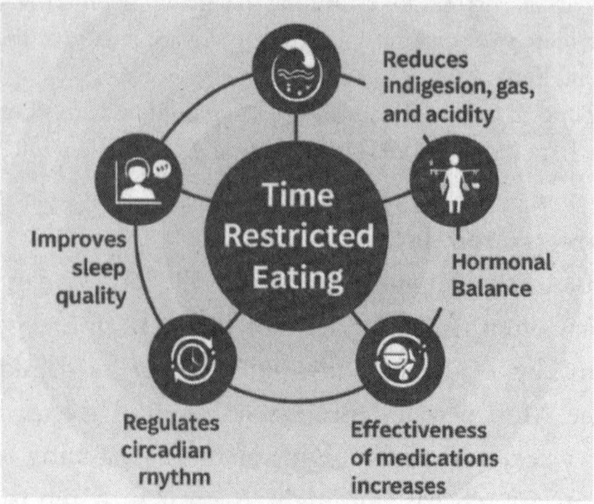

Image 8.2: *Time-restricted eating*

> **What is metabolism?**
>
> The food we eat gets converted into energy in our body. This process is called metabolism. Think of it as a small kitchen inside your body. Whatever food you eat goes into this kitchen, and there it is converted into energy—the fuel that helps you walk, talk and work. If this kitchen works well, your body functions smoothly. But if it slows down, you feel tired, gain weight and don't digest food properly.
>
> That's why eating balanced meals, staying active and getting good sleep are very important for a healthy metabolism.

Reading this, it might feel like I'm promoting fasting, but that's not the case. Not everyone needs to do fasting or intermittent fasting. What's important is that we should not overload our body with food when it is in a 'shutdown mode'. As we saw earlier, if we eat when the body is not ready to digest, that food often gets stored directly as fat. Research has shown that giving our digestive system a proper 'resting phase' is very important for maintaining hormonal balance.

Eat Minimally Processed, Whole Foods—and Read Labels Carefully

This may sound very simple, but in today's world, we end up eating a lot of *highly processed foods*—not always by choice, but often without even realising it. Some common but 'hidden' processed foods include ketchup, cheese, instant noodles, biscuits (including rusk), breakfast cereals, namkeen, ready-to-eat meals, sandwich spreads, bread, ready-to-cook spice mixes, instant breakfast mixes…and the list can go on.

In a busy lifestyle, it may not be practical (or affordable) to cook everything from scratch or eat only organic foods.

A practical rule of thumb is: limit highly processed foods to no more than three items a day.

A not-so-fun (scary) fact: Children are at the highest risk of being exposed to ultra-processed foods!

It's also important to remember that not every packaged food is unhealthy. If we assume so, then we'd be left only with raw fruits and vegetables—because even something as basic as wheat flour comes in a packet nowadays.

Let's break it down:

1. **Unprocessed or minimally processed foods:**
   Whole fruits, vegetables, cut veggies, salad leaves, eggs, meat, marinated chicken, milk, oils, flour, and so on. These foods are processed only for safety or hygiene (like milk pasteurization, oil extraction). Such foods are safe and healthy.
2. **Processed foods:**
   Commercially prepared, but with recognisable ingredients. Examples: bread, marinated meat or chicken, canned fruits, tomato purée, spice blends, idli-dosa batter, cheese, paneer, etc. These foods can be part of a healthy diet when chosen wisely. For example, packaged paneer is still a good protein source because it hasn't been altered much.
3. **Ultra-processed foods:**
   These undergo multiple processes like pulping, molding, extrusion, frying, and so on. They are designed to be *hyper-palatable* (very tasty and hard to resist) and to last longer on shelves. But in the process, many nutrients are lost and replaced with artificial additives such as propylene glycol, emulsifiers, anti-caking agents, artificial colours, sodium nitrites, and more—ingredients most of us can't even pronounce or visualise.

Examples of ultra-processed foods

Fruit juice drinks, carbonated soft drinks, candies, chocolates, biscuits, ready-to-eat snacks, frosted breakfast cereals, energy bars, instant noodles, chocolate spreads, chips, mock meat, heat-and-eat frozen meals, and so on.

Remember: These products often carry claims like 'natural', '100% whole', or 'fortified with vitamins and minerals'. But in reality, they are far from healthy. Compared to their natural form, ultra-processed foods contain more calories and additives, and are designed to be addictive—'once you eat one, you'll want more'. That's what makes them a serious health risk.

You might feel you don't eat too many of these. But let's look at a very common day's diet:

- Morning: 1 cup tea + 4 'high-fibre' digestive biscuits
- Breakfast: Chocolate-flavoured cereal, 1 glass packaged fruit juice, 2 toasts with low-fat bread spread
- Mid-morning snack: Low-sugar packaged energy bar
- Lunch: 2 rotis, some sabzi, 1 chocolate
- Tea-time: Grilled sandwich with processed cheese and mayonnaise
- Dinner: Instant noodles with cola
- Dessert: Ice cream
- This seemingly 'normal' day actually contains 8+ ultra-processed foods. That's why a realistic and healthy target is: limit ultra-processed foods to no more than three items per day.

But how do you actually do this?

1. Learn to read nutrition labels. When you understand what's really going into your food, you can make better choices.

2. Cook more at home. Homemade meals are the true key to health.
3. Choose house parties or potlucks over eating out. When food is made at home, you have more control over what you're eating.
4. Eat with family or friends instead of alone and in front of the TV.
5. Plan your meals for the week in advance. When you already know what's coming up, you're less likely to reach for junk food.
6. Stock up on healthy options and clear processed foods from your kitchen. If it's not in the house, the chances of eating it drop by 70 per cent!
7. Include at least three different colours on your plate. This ensures you eat a more varied and nutrient-rich diet.
8. Eat something before grocery shopping. Shopping on an empty stomach increases the chances of buying processed foods.
9. Choose movie or show times after meals. This helps avoid popcorn or other junk snacks.
10. Keep attractive bottles for homemade drinks. You'll be more likely to enjoy healthy homemade beverages.
11. Keep healthy food visible and accessible. For example, a banana on your desk is more likely to be eaten, but if it's tucked away in the kitchen, you might forget about it!

How to read nutrition labels

1. Ignore the front-of-pack claims.
2. Always check the back of the package.
3. Look at the ingredients list.
4. If any ingredient you're trying to avoid is in the top 3, skip the product.
   Example 1: People with diabetes should avoid added sugar, excess salt or corn starch.
   Example 2: If instant soup lists potato starch as the first ingredient, it's basically a hidden form of sugar.
5. Check the order of ingredients carefully.
   Ingredients are listed in descending order by weight. The first 3 are the main ingredients.
   Example 1: Jam with ingredients listed as sugar, 46% fruit purée, thickener → more than 50 per cent sugar.
   Example 2: If you buy 'wholewheat' pasta but whole wheat isn't the first ingredient, it's not truly wholewheat.
6. Identify hidden trans fats and sugars.
   Example: High fructose corn syrup is a common hidden sugar linked to diabetes and obesity.[23]

Raw vs. cooked food

Some people believe that anything raw is always the best. But in reality, for most vegetables, nutrients become more bioavailable (easier for the body to absorb) when they are cooked or steamed.

From a nutritionist's perspective

What matters more is that you are eating enough vegetables, not whether they're raw or cooked. Always look at the bigger picture. If having spinach as soup or stuffed in a paratha helps you eat more of it, then go ahead and eat it that way without guilt!

Here's a simple guideline I follow:

- **Leafy greens:** Steamed or lightly sautéed works well. For example, methi paratha with mint chutney, amla pickle, carrot salad or kachumber with a squeeze of lemon.
- **Colourful veggies:** Carrot, sweet potato, pumpkin, yam—best when steamed.
- **Tomatoes:** Cooking enhances lycopene (an antioxidant), making them more beneficial.
- **Fruits:** Always best eaten raw.
- **Non-vegetarian foods:** Easier to digest when cooked.

Food convenience

With our busy lifestyles, we often need to take shortcuts while cooking. I'd love to extract fresh coconut milk myself, but most days I don't have the time, willpower, or even the know-how to do it. That's why we turn to convenient options like ready-to-use coconut milk. Making life easier is not wrong, whether it's using coconut milk from a tetra pack or can, tomato purée, frozen peas, corn kernels or pre-cut vegetables. The main thing is you're still cooking at home, which is already a big win for your health.

But don't forget to check nutrition labels. Tomato purée should list only tomatoes. Coconut milk should be just coconut milk, without stabilisers, thickeners or emulsifiers.

Frozen fruits and vegetables are also very convenient. Just remember: freezing can reduce vitamin C by up to 50 per cent.[4] That's why it's important to include vitamin C-rich foods like lemon juice in your meals.

When using pre-cut or cleaned vegetables, eat them within 48 hours of the packing date. Once fruits are cut, oxidation starts, and Vitamin C is the first nutrient to degrade. Squeezing a little lemon juice on them helps. If pre-cut veggies need to be stored longer, it's better to freeze them than keep them in the fridge.

Food pairing is important too

Even food and nutrients have their own 'partners'! Fat-soluble vitamins like vitamins A, D, E and K are better absorbed by the body when eaten with fat-rich foods. For example, if you eat carrots, pumpkin, spinach, eggs or mushrooms with a little oil, butter, ghee, coconut oil or coconut, your body can absorb their benefits more effectively.

Similarly, iron-rich foods are best absorbed when paired with vitamin C, which helps 'release' iron from food and also blocks substances that interfere with iron absorption. So, if you're eating spinach, drumsticks, meat, eggs or beetroot, add lemon, orange, amchur (dry mango powder) or amla alongside. On the other hand, avoid calcium-rich foods like milk or yogurt at the same time, because calcium reduces iron absorption. For example, if your child eats iron-fortified cornflakes with milk for breakfast, try giving them some pomegranate seeds or spinach later in the day to balance absorption.

Finally, don't overthink cooking methods or combinations. If you are eating home-cooked meals, you are already a big step ahead for good health.

A little better—every time

Perfection is just an idea; progress should be our real focus.

When we decide to 'eat healthy' or 'get fit', we often try to make too many big changes overnight. The mindset of 'all or nothing'. Like 'If I can't eat perfectly, I may as well give up' often becomes the biggest hurdle in reaching our goals.

I've seen this with many of my clients. At the start, they feel that unless every single meal is perfect, unless they exercise daily, follow a 100 per cent balanced diet, and get perfect sleep, they've achieved nothing. But that's not how our body and mind work.

If we focus on making just one thing a little better each time, it becomes easier to sustain those habits and gradually build on them.

Take Neha, for example, a busy working woman. Her rising blood sugar levels and increasing diabetes medications made her realise that unless she made changes now, serious health problems were just around the corner.

Being hardworking and ambitious, she decided she would cook all her meals at home, join the gym and lose 6–7 kilograms in a month.

Day 1 went perfectly. She cooked, exercised and felt proud. But on Day 2, her cook didn't show up. She couldn't go to the gym, made herself breakfast, but skipped lunch due to work pressure. By evening, she was exhausted and ordered food online. She felt like a complete failure.

When she came to me, she said, 'Tell me a simple, sustainable way to eat healthy, something I can do for life.' I told her, 'Pick the easiest option. What can you definitely do every day? Choose the simplest change.'[5]

She replied, 'I can get up early and go to the gym, I've paid a lot of money and don't want it to go to waste.' So, we started there. That week, her only focus was to go to the gym four times. Anything more was a bonus. She ended up going five times—and was thrilled.

The next week, I asked her to add just one healthy home-cooked meal. She chose breakfast, her favourite. Six days of nutritious breakfasts plus regular workouts helped her lose half a kilo more, and she felt satisfied and confident.

Start small and simple. If you can change everything overnight, great—but in reality, that rarely happens. It's far easier to build one habit at a time and then layer new ones on top, rather than overhaul your entire system at once.[6]

Even if you're so busy that you can't manage a full breakfast, starting with just one boiled egg still counts as progress.

James Clear notes in *Atomic Habits*, 'You do not rise to the level of your goals. You fall to the level of your systems.' That's why, every time, just a little better.

If you set goals that are achievable every single day, you'll find it much easier to sustain healthy eating and fitness habits in the long run.

Pay attention to your own body. Whether you're following a diet plan given by a nutritionist, a meal plan suggested by your gym trainer, or your own 'clean eating' programme, it's crucial to listen to your body's signals. If your health is truly improving (and here I don't mean just 'fine', I mean genuinely healthy), your body will show it in the following ways:

1. **Your energy levels will improve:**
   Energy and nutrition are closely linked. For example, if you're not getting enough B-complex vitamins like B1 and B12, even while on a diet, you may experience fatigue, sluggishness and lack of motivation to work.
2. **Your face will glow and hair will stay healthy:**
   Your skin is a reflection of your health. If your face looks dull, your cheeks are sunken, and your hands and feet

are very dry, it's a sign that your body is not in a truly healthy state. Many weight-loss diets reduce weight but can increase hair fall. If you notice this happening, it's important to make immediate adjustments to your diet.

3. **Your digestion will improve:**
   Yes! If you're eating properly and in a balanced way, you shouldn't experience constipation, frequent bloating, bad breath or repeated trips to the bathroom for gas. One of the first signs that your health is improving is better digestion. If you previously didn't have constipation but now do, or if you find yourself relying on frequent laxatives after starting a diet, it's a clear signal that serious changes are needed in what and how you're eating.
4. **You'll feel full and satisfied:**
   Remember that 'Hangry kya?' ('Are you hangry?') ad? It's true! Hunger can make you irritable, impatient and short-tempered. If your friends or family have been saying, 'You've been so cranky lately,' trust me, the reason could be **what** you're eating...or not eating! When you eat in a way that leaves you satisfied, that's a true sign of good health.
5. **Your sleep improves:**
   Sleep and the body's repair processes are closely linked to what you eat. Have you ever eaten a heavy meal like biryani, with lots of gravy, and then struggled to sleep all night, worried about acidity or food reflux? That's why sometimes we avoid eating healthily. Even going to bed hungry doesn't guarantee good sleep. Remember, if your food isn't letting you sleep well, it's not right for you.
6. **Your clothes will fit better (looser or sometimes tighter!)**:
   The weighing scale is not always the best measure of progress. When you eat healthily and exercise, you'll

notice your clothes fitting better. For example, a blouse that felt too tight might now feel more comfortable, or pants you couldn't button before might fit easily. Sometimes, a shirt may feel snug around your arms, but that's usually because of increased muscle growth. This is a positive sign of improvement!

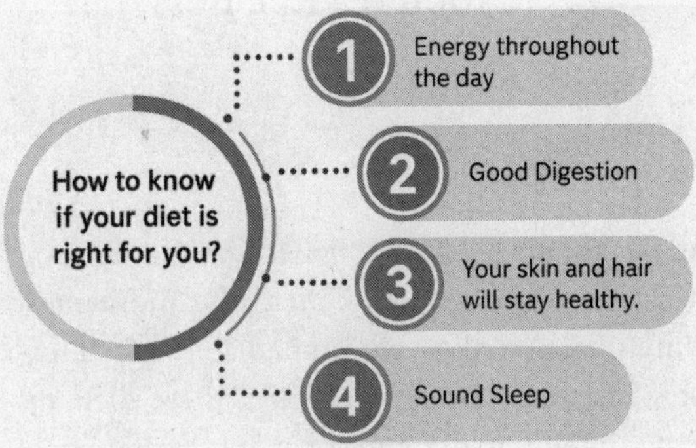

Image 8.3: *Key markers of a well-balanced diet*

9

'Fad Diets', Different Names, Same Principle: Eat Less

Nowadays, there's a strong belief that to improve your health, you need to go on a diet. The moment we hear the name of a new diet, we immediately ask, 'How much weight will I lose?' But the truth is, these diets may have different names, but the core principle is always the same, eat less than your body needs, i.e., create a calorie deficit.

Now, if someone directly said 'eat less to lose weight', it wouldn't sound very appealing. So, a wall of imagination and fancy words is built around it, giving rise to Keto, OMAD, zero-fat diets, or 'eat 45 minutes in the morning and 45 minutes in the evening' type plans.

Do the names change the principle?

No. The principle remains the same: 'Eat less, lose weight.'

OMAD: One meal a day

OMAD stands for 'one meal a day'. Again, the goal is a calorie deficit. Often, this single meal doesn't provide enough protein, fibre or essential vitamins. Over time, the body starts losing muscle, constant fatigue sets in, and instead of weight stabilising, it often rebounds. Psychologically, the constant thought of 'only one meal a day' can disturb one's relationship with food. Eating disorders often start this way.

Keto diet: Saying goodbye to carbs

In the keto diet, carbohydrates are almost completely eliminated. You can't eat regular roti or rice, and even vegetables are limited because they contain some carbs. What remains are fats and proteins. Without carbs, the body produces ketones from fat for energy—this is the concept of ketosis. Weight drops quickly at first, but this is largely water loss. Within a few days, issues can appear—from constipation[1] and hair fall to mental unease and hormonal imbalance. Consistently maintaining keto is only possible for very few people; if stopped, weight usually comes back.

Zero-fat diet: Is fat really the enemy?

In this diet, all fats are forbidden—ghee, oil, peanuts, nuts—everything. But fat isn't just 'fat'; it's essential for hormone production, brain function, skin and hair health, and reproductive well-being. A lack of fat can lead to hormonal imbalance, irregular periods, hair fall, dry skin, and on top of that, a persistent low mood. In these diets, they even tell you to add a tempering of water and spices to your food. Basically, taking the joy out of your meals along with the fat!

Forty-five-minute two-meal diet

This approach tells you to eat whatever you want but only twice a day, within fixed 45-minute windows. The idea is that the body releases less insulin, so weight will drop. But again, what's really happening is that limiting meals to two times a day creates a calorie deficit. No one pays attention to what you eat in those two meals—whether there's enough protein, fibre or nutrients. While some people may find this simple, for many, especially women, this method is insufficient for energy, hormones and muscles.

Once your body realises it could face another famine, it starts storing more energy. This is the reason behind yo-yo dieting—weight drops, you stop, it comes back, you diet again, it comes back again…

If you want to break this cycle, there's only one answer.

Balanced. Sustainable. Wise.

- Ask yourself: Can the diet you follow work for every stage of your life?
- Don't pay the price of your body just to lose weight. Losing muscle, bones, periods or energy for a slim figure is a very expensive 'loss'.
- Diet is not a trend, it's a lifestyle. And changing your diet doesn't just mean 'eat less', it means 'eat in balanced amounts'.
- The final takeaway: 'Diets never last, habits do.'

10

Finally, Let's Sit Down to Eat!

In this book, I've explained *what to eat, how much to eat, and how to eat it* in a scientific yet simple way. And yes, there's no preachy 'don't eat this' tone anywhere. Because in my view, health is **not a punishment, it's a habit**.

Here, we've explored the five main components of diet. I've presented their uses, roles and what happens when we overdo them—all in a straightforward and honest manner. They are as follows:

- **Protein**: The foundation of the body. Muscles, heart, brain, hair, skin—they're all made of protein
- **Fibre**: Essential for digestion, blood sugar control, and preventing constipation
- **Fats**: Choosing healthy fats supports everything from hormones to brain function
- **Carbs:** Provide energy that keeps your body running, but the type and quantity matter
- **Micronutrients:** Vitamins and minerals that are small in quantity but crucial for life

And I've shown how to build your ideal balanced plate: **50 per cent vegetables, 25 per cent protein, and 25 per cent grains.**

See? Simple!

Feeling a little overwhelmed after reading everything is natural. But remember, this isn't difficult, it's just outside your usual habits. I've never suggested any specific food brands, exotic superfoods or drastic diet changes. On the contrary, I've focused on creating a healthy diet using what's easily available at home, in your tradition and in your local market.

For example:

- Matki, moong, lentils: these are our protein banks.
- Pithla-bhakri, thalipeeth, khichdi: these are sources of whole grains.
- Vegetables: whatever is available. There's no need to go hunting for exotic or English vegetables.

What's on your plate is already nutritious—you just need to adjust the quantities a little.

Can a single plate be healthy?

Yes. And even if it's not 'Instagram-worthy', that plate can shape your health for the future. Healthy eating doesn't mean making huge changes. It just requires a little thought: 'Does my plate have protein today?', 'Is there fibre?', 'Does my plate look colorful?', etc.

This book is 'the key in your hands'

Through this book, I've given you the key to unlock your diet. The answers to your questions about weight, diabetes, fatigue, hair fall, digestion, and everything else are hidden in a well-planned and thoughtful diet. My goal isn't just to give you a formula, but to give you a way of thinking.

Trends might change tomorrow, but once you develop the habit of thinking, you'll always be able to decide whether any diet is truly right for you.

Final advice: don't rush while eating, and even less while making decisions

- Before trying something new, ask yourself: does this really serve me, or is it just advertising?
- The maths of health doesn't run on 'calories', it runs on balance.
- And yes, meals aren't just about the body. They're about our culture, our care and our memories. Enjoy them as such.

And now?

The book is ending, and you might be hungry. Go on, open the fridge. Pick two vegetables from what's available. Are you going to make dal-rice or a 2-egg omelette?

And don't forget: eat calmly, with your phone away. Because achieving health isn't a race. It's about pausing, understanding and then choosing.

See you again, on your plate and in your thoughts!

Acknowledgements

This book has been five years in the making: five years of research, writing, rewriting, questioning and refining. And while my name sits on the cover, this work would not exist without the collective effort, patience and faith of so many incredible people.

First, to Manish Khurana at Bloomsbury Publications, thank you for believing in this book from the very beginning and for your editorial wisdom. To my literary agent Saksham Garg, thank you for championing this project and for being the bridge between my vision and the world that needed to read it.

To my brilliant team—Shreya, Aishwarya, Gauri, Madhura, Reiza, Himani, and Dipali—you were the backbone of this entire process. The research, the planning, the iterations, the illustrations—you showed up for this book with dedication and heart. I am deeply grateful.

Krish Ashok, Dr Tanaya Narendra, and CA Rachana Ranade, thank you for your generous endorsements. Your voices carry weight, and your support means the world to me.

Omkar Jadhav and Viraj Pawar, thank you for helping create a cover that captures exactly what this book stands for—simple, honest, and rooted.

To my family and friends, thank you for understanding the endless evenings and weekends I disappeared into writing. Forforgiving my absence and quietly holding space for me to do this work.

And finally, to Dhruv and my son Raajas—you are my constant. Dhruv, thank you for being my sounding board, my anchor, and my unwavering support. Raajas, this book is dedicated to you. Everything I write, I write hoping to leave behind a world where you, and everyone else, can eat with clarity, confidence, and joy and be healthy.

Notes

Introduction

1 Agnihotri, A., '27 year old woman weighing just 22 kilograms dies after following extreme "fruitarian" diet; Manipal doctors warn about dangers', *Hindustan Times*, 9 October 2025, https://www.hindustantimes.com/lifestyle/health/27-year-old-woman-dies-after-following-extreme-fruitarian-diet-weighing-just-22-kg-manipal-doctors-warn-about-risks-101759988135967.html.

2 'Vegan influencer "starved to death," friends say', *New York Post*, 31 July 2023, July 31, https://nypost.com/2023/07/31/vegan-influencer-starved-to-death-friends/.

3 Clarance, D., 'US man bizarrely leaks cholesterol from his body. It was due to his diet', *India Today*, 25 January 2025, https://www.indiatoday.in/health/story/us-man-bizarrely-leaks-cholesterol-from-his-body-diet-2669669-2025-01-25.

1. Protein Is Like God!

1 'A Brief Note on Nutrient Requirements for Indians, the Recommended Dietary Allowances (RDA) and the Estimated Average Requirements (EAR)', ICMR -NIN, 2020. (n.d.), retrieved 24 September 2025, https-//www.nin.res.in/rdabook/brief_note.pdf.

2 Weijs, P. J. M., 'Protein requirement in obesity', *Current Opinion in Clinical Nutrition and Metabolic Care,* 28 (1): 27–32, 2025, https://doi.org/10.1097/MCO.0000000000001087.

3 Bray, G. A., et al., 'Effect of dietary protein content on weight gain, energy expenditure, and body composition during overeating: A randomized controlled trial', *JAMA* 307(1): 47–55, 2012, https://doi.org/10.1001/jama.2011.1918.

4 Pomeroy, E., et al., 'Ancient origins of low lean mass among South Asians and implications for modern type 2 diabetes susceptibility', *Scientific Reports* 9(1): 105–15, 2019, https://doi.org/10.1038/s41598-019-46960-9.

5 Raubenheimer, D., and S.J. Simpson, 'Protein appetite as an integrator in the obesity system: the protein leverage hypothesis', Philosophical Transactions of the Royal Society of London, Series B*, Biological Sciences* 378 (1888): 202202–12, 2023, https://doi.org/10.1098/rstb.2022.0212.

6 Zibellini, J., et al, 'Effect of diet-induced weight loss on muscle strength in adults with overweight or obesity: a systematic review and meta-analysis of clinical trials', *Obesity Reviews* 17(8): 647–63, 2016, https://doi.org/10.1111/obr.12422.

7 Peters, S.A.E., S.H. Bots, and M. Woodward, 'Sex differences in the association between measures of general and central adiposity and the risk of myocardial infarction: Results from the UK Biobank', *Journal of the American Heart Association* 7(5), e008507, 2018, https-//doi.org/10.1161/JAHA.117.008507.

8 'A Brief Note on Nutrient Requirements for Indians, the Recommended Dietary Allowances (RDA) and the Estimated Average Requirements (EAR)', *ICMR-NIN*, 2020. (n.d.), https://www.nin.res.in/rdabook/brief_note.pdf, retrieved 24 September 2025.

9 'Source: Adapted from Clinical Guidelines on the Identification, Evaluation, and Treatment of Overweight and Obesity in Adults: The Evidence Report', 2022, https://www.nhlbi.nih.gov/sites/default/files/media/docs/bmi_tbl.pdf.

10 Kang, Jung Hyun, Z. Dong, and Seung Ho Shin, 'Benefits of Soybean in the Era of Precision Medicine- A Review of Clinical Evidence', *Journal of Microbiology and Biotechnology* 33(12): 1552–62, 2023, https://doi.org/10.4014/jmb.2308.08016.

11 International Institute for Population Sciences (IIPS) and ICF, *National Family Health Survey (NFHS-5),* 2019–21: India, 2021.

12 Clarke, R., et al., 'Dietary lipids and blood cholesterol: quantitative meta-analysis of metabolic ward studies', *BMJ* 314(7074): 112, 1997, https://doi.org/10.1136/bmj.314.7074.112.

13 These blood tests can show if your protein intake is enough, but not everyone needs to get them done. Albumin is a protein that carries nutrients in your blood, globulin helps fight infections, and the A/G ratio shows the balance between them.

14 Qiao, K., et al., 'The evaluation of yeast protein quality as a new and sustainable source of dietary protein', *Journal of Agricultural and Food Chemistry* 73(38): 24127–38, 2025, https://doi.org/10.1021/acs.jafc.5c06807

15 Wu, G., 'Dietary Protein Intake and Human Health', *Food & Function* 7(3): 1251–65, 2016, https://doi.org/10.1039/c5fo01530h. 5 scoops of protein = 120 g protein, which, in turn, amounts to 2 g protein/kg of body weight for a 60 kg adult.

16 Schoenfeld, B., et al., 'The effect of protein timing on muscle strength and hypertrophy: A meta-analysis', *Journal of the International Society of Sports Nutrition* 10(1), Article 53, 2013, https://doi.org/10.1186/1550-2783-10-53.

17 Ko, G.-J., et al., 'The effects of high-protein diets on kidney health and longevity', *Journal of the American Society of Nephrology* 31(8): 1667–79, 2020, https://doi.org/10.1681/ASN.2020010028.

18 Korovljev, D., et al., 'The effects of 8-week creatine hydrochloride and creatine ethyl ester supplementation on cognition, clinical outcomes, and brain creatine levels in perimenopausal and menopausal women (CONCRET-MENOPA): A randomized controlled trial', *Journal of the American Nutrition Association,* 1–12, 2025, https://doi.org/10.1080/27697061.2025.2551184.

19 Antonio, J., et al., 'Common questions and misconceptions about creatine supplementation: What does the scientific evidence really show?', *Journal of the International Society of Sports Nutrition* 18(1), 13, 2021, https://doi.org/10.1186/s12970-021-00412-w.

20 Lak, M., et al., 'Does creatine cause hair loss? A 12-week randomized controlled trial', *Journal of the International Society of Sports Nutrition* 22(sup1), 2495229, 2025, https://doi.org/10.1080/15502783.2025.2495229

21 Wang, Z., et al., 'Effects of Creatine Supplementation and Resistance Training on Muscle Strength Gains in Adults <50 Years of Age: A Systematic Review and Meta-Analysis', *Nutrients* 16(21): 3665, 2024, https://doi.org/10.3390/nu16213665.

22 Wax, B., et al., 'Creatine for Exercise and Sports Performance, with Recovery Considerations for Healthy Populations', *Nutrients* 13(6): 1915, 2021, https://doi.org/10.3390/nu13061915.

2 Fibre

1 Xie, W., et al., 'The burden of colorectal cancer attributable to diet low in fiber from 1990 to 2019: A global, regional and national analysis', *The Journal of Nutrition, Health & Aging* 26(12): 1061–69, 2022, https://doi.org/10.1007/s12603-022-1865-x.

2 Nucci, D., et al., 'Association between dietary fibre intake and colorectal adenoma: A systematic review and meta-analysis', *International Journal of Environmental Research and Public Health* 18(8): 4168, 2021, https://doi.org/10.3390/ijerph18084168.

3 Sreemathy V, and Triveni K., 'Assessment of Dietary Fiber Intake in Adults: Consideration of Gender and Age Disparities', *J Clin Biomed Sci 2024* 14(3): 85-90, 2021, https://doi.org/10.58739/jcbs/v14i3.108.

4 Farooqui, A.A., 'Importance and roles of fiber in the diet', in A.A. Farooqui (ed.), *High-calorie diet and the human brain*, Springer, 2015, pp. 193–218, https://doi.org/10.1007/978-3-319-15254-7.

5 Lu, K., et al., 'Effect of viscous soluble dietary fiber on glucose and lipid metabolism in patients with type 2 diabetes mellitus: a systematic review and meta-analysis on randomized clinical trials', *Frontiers in Nutrition* 10, Article 1253312, 2023, https://doi.org/10.3389/fnut.2023.1253312.

6 Park, Y., et al., 'Dietary fiber intake and risk of colorectal cancer: a pooled analysis of prospective cohort studies', *JAMA* 294(22): 2849–57, 2005, https://doi.org/10.1001/jama.294.22.2849.

7 Soliman, G. A., 'Dietary fiber, atherosclerosis, and cardiovascular disease', *Nutrients* 11(5): 1155, 2019, https://doi.org/10.3390/nu11051155.

8 Guan, Z. W., E.-Z. Yu, and Q. Feng, 'Soluble Dietary Fiber, One of the Most Important Nutrients for the Gut Microbiota', *Molecules* 26(22): 6802, 2021, https://doi.org/10.3390/molecules26226802.

9 La Torre, D., K. Verbeke, and B. Dalile, 'Dietary fibre and the gut–brain axis: microbiota-dependent and independent mechanisms of action', *Gut Microbiome* 2, e3, 2021, https://doi.org/10.1017/gmb.2021.3.

10 Triffoni-Melo, A. T., et al., 'HIGH-FIBER DIET PROMOTES METABOLIC, HORMONAL, AND SATIETY EFFECTS IN OBESE WOMEN ON A SHORT-TERM CALORIC RESTRICTION', *Arquivos de Gastroenterologia* 60(2): 163–71, 2023, https://doi.org/10.1590/s0004-2803.202302022-96.

11 Dwijayanti, A., and A.P. Darlian, 'The importance of dietary fiber on stress hormone in pregnancy: A literature review', *Jurnal Optimasi Sistem Industri* 20(1): 1–6, 2021. (Dietary fiber and cortisol balance)

12 Wang, X., et al., 'Dietary modulation of the enteric nervous system: From molecular mechanisms to therapeutic applications', *Nutrients* 17(22): 3519, 2025, https://doi.org/10.3390/nu17223519.

13 Ghoshal, U. C., et al., 'Indian consensus on chronic constipation in adults: A joint position statement of the Indian Motility and Functional Diseases Association and the Indian Society of Gastroenterology', *Indian Journal of Gastroenterology* 37(6): 526–44, 2018, https://doi.org/10.1007/s12664-018-0894-1.

14 Staller, K., et al., 'Chronic constipation as a risk factor for colorectal cancer: results from a nationwide, case-control study', *Clinical Gastroenterology and Hepatology* 20(8): 1867–76, e2, 2022, https://doi.org/10.1016/j.cgh.2021.10.024.

15 Celiberto, F., et al., 'Fibres and colorectal cancer: Clinical and molecular evidence', *International Journal of Molecular Sciences* 24(17), 13501, 2023, https://doi.org/10.3390/ijms241713501.

16 O'Keefe, S.J., 'The association between dietary fibre deficiency and high-income lifestyle-associated diseases: Burkitt's hypothesis revisited', *The Lancet Gastroenterology & Hepatology* 4(12): 984–96, 2019, https://doi.org/10.1016/S2468-1253(19)30257-2.
17 National Institute of Nutrition, 'Indian Food Composition Tables', Indian Council of Medical Research, Department of Health Research, Ministry of Health and Family Welfare, Government of India, 2017.
18 Wang, Z., et al., 'Psyllium husk powder improves constipation by remodeling gut microbiota and improving intestinal metabolites', *Food Bioscience* 64, 105828, 2025, https://doi.org/10.1016/j.fbio.2025.105828.
19 Hassan, Z.A.H., et al., 'Dietary fiber and glycolipid metabolism: Insights from molecular mechanisms and targeted interventions', *Nutrients* 17(22): 3521, 2025, https://doi.org/10.3390/nu17223521.
20 Ma, Y., 'Single-component versus multicomponent dietary goals for the metabolic syndrome: A randomized trial', *Annals of Internal Medicine* 162(4): 317–27, 2015, https://doi.org/10.7326/M14-0611.
21 'Revised Short Summary Report-2024', ICMR-NIN Expert Group on Nutrient Requirements for Indians, Recommended Dietary Allowances (RDA) and Estimated Average Requirements (EAR)-2020.
22 Hu, X., et al., 'Modification of potato starch by using superheated steam', *Carbohydrate Polymers* 198, 375–84, 2018, https://doi.org/10.1016/j.carbpol.2018.06.110.

3 Fats

1 Chang, C.Y., D.S. Ke, and J.Y. Chen, 'Essential fatty acids and human brain', *Acta Neurologica Taiwanica* 18(4): 231–41, 2009, https://pubmed.ncbi.nlm.nih.gov/20329590/.
2 Ziomkiewicz, A., et al., 'Body fat, energy balance and estradiol levels: A study based on hormonal profiles from complete menstrual cycles', *Human Reproduction* 23(11): 2555–63, 2008, https://doi.org/10.1093/humrep/den213.

3 Liu, X., M. Gong, and N. Wu, 'Research progress on the relationship between free fatty acid profile and type 2 diabetes complicated by coronary heart disease', *Frontiers in Endocrinology* 15, Article 1503704, 2024, https://doi.org/10.3389/fendo.2024.1503704.

4 Centres for Disease Control and Prevention, 'Heart disease risk factors', 2 December 2024, https://www.cdc.gov/heart-disease/risk-factors/index.html.

5 Mazza, E., et al., 'Obesity, dietary patterns, and hormonal balance modulation: Gender-specific impacts', *Nutrients* 16(11): 1629, 2024, https://doi.org/10.3390/nu16111629.

6 Yang, J. J., et al., 'Dietary fat intake and lung cancer risk: A pooled analysis', *Journal of Clinical Oncology* 35(26): 3055–64, 2017, https://doi.org/10.1200/JCO.2017.73.3329.

7 Carroll, K.K., 'Dietary fats and cancer', *American Journal of Clinical Nutrition* 53(4, Suppl): 1064S–1067S, 1991, https://doi.org/10.1093/ajcn/53.4.1064S.

8 Guasch-Ferré, Marta, et al., 'Consumption of Olive Oil and Risk of Total and Cause-Specific Mortality among U.S. Adults', *Journal of the American College of Cardiology* 79(2): 101–112, 18 January 2022, https://doi.org/10.1016/j.jacc.2021.10.041.

9 Schwingshackl, L., and G. Hoffmann, 'Monounsaturated fatty acids and risk of cardiovascular disease: Synopsis of the evidence available from systematic reviews and meta-analyses', *Nutrients* 4(12): 1989–2007, 2012, https://doi.org/10.3390/nu4121989.

10 Zock, P. L., and M.B. Katan, 'Hydrogenation alternatives: Effects of trans fatty acids and stearic acid versus linoleic acid on serum lipids and lipoproteins in humans', *Journal of Lipid Research* 33(3): 399–410, 1992, https://doi.org/10.1016/S0022-2275(20)38255-7.

11 Mauger, J. F., et al., 'Effect of different forms of dietary hydrogenated fats on LDL particle size and cardiovascular risk markers', *The American Journal of Clinical Nutrition*, Advance online publication, 2022, https://doi.org/10.1016/S0002-9165(22)33196.

12 Sudheendran, S., C.C. Chang, and R.J. Deckelbaum, 'N-3 vs. saturated fatty acids: Effects on the arterial wall', *Prostaglandins, Leukotrienes and Essential Fatty Acids* 82(4-6): 205–209, 2010, https://doi.org/10.1016/j.plefa.2010.02.020.

13 Zeng, Wei, et al. "Reassessing the Effects of Dietary Fat on Cardiovascular Disease in China: A Review of the Last Three Decades', *Nutrients* 15(19): 4214, 29 September 2023, https://doi.org/10.3390/nu15194214.

14 Bray, G. A., & Popkin, B. M. (1998). Dietary fat intake does affect obesity! *The American Journal of Clinical Nutrition,* 68(6), 1157–1173. https://doi.org/10.1093/ajcn/68.6.1157

15 World Health Organization. (2025, June 3). *Healthy diet* [Fact sheet]. https://www.who.int/news-room/fact-sheets/detail/healthy-diet

16 Zhang, Y., Zhuang, P., Wu, F., He, W., Mao, L., Jia, W., Zhang, Y., Chen, X., & Jiao, J. (2021). Cooking oil/fat consumption and deaths from cardiometabolic diseases and other causes: prospective analysis of 521,120 individuals. *BMC Medicine,* 19(1). https://doi.org/10.1186/s12916-021-01961-2

17 Ministry of Consumer Affairs, Food & Public Distribution. (n.d.), *Vanaspati – Consumer products*, Government of India, https://consumeraffairs.gov.in/public/upload/admin/cmsfiles/consumer_products/Vanaspati_consumer_products.pdf.

18 Grzelczyk, J., J. Oracz, and I. Gałązka-Czarnecka,'Quality assessment of waste from olive oil production and design of biodegradable packaging', *Foods* 11(23): 3776, 2022, https://doi.org/10.3390/foods11233776.

19 Hewlings, S.,'Coconuts and health: Different chain lengths of saturated fats require different consideration', *Journal of Cardiovascular Development and Disease* 7(4): 59, 2020, https://doi.org/10.3390/jcdd7040059.

20 Mohammadi Hosseinabadi, Susan, and Javad Nasrollahzadeh, 'Effects of Diets Rich in Ghee or Olive Oil on Cardiometabolic Risk Factors in Healthy Adults: A 2-Period, Crossover, Randomized Trial', *British Journal of Nutrition,* 1–30, 19 November 2021, https://doi.org/10.1017/s0007114521004645.

21 Froyen, Erik, and Bonny Burns-Whitmore, 'The Effects of Linoleic Acid Consumption on Lipid Risk Markers for Cardiovascular Disease in Healthy Individuals: A Review of Human Intervention Trials', *Nutrients* 12(8): 2329, 4 August 2020, https://doi.org/10.3390/nu12082329.

22 Ministry of Consumer Affairs, Food & Public Distribution. 'Vanaspati – Consumer products', Government of India, https://consumeraffairs.gov.in/public/upload/admin/cmsfiles/consumer_products/Vanaspati_consumer_products.pdf.

23 Hashemian, M., et al., 'Red meat consumption and risk of non-alcoholic fatty liver disease and non-alcoholic steatohepatitis: a systematic review', *Journal of Translational Internal Medicine* 9(3): 123–130, 2021, https://doi.org/10.2478/jtim-2021-0023.

24 Chueire, V. B., and E. Muscelli, E., 'Effect of free fatty acids on insulin secretion, insulin sensitivity and incretin effect – a narrative review', Archives of Endocrinology and Metabolism 65(1): 24–31, 2021, https://doi.org/10.20945/2359-3997000000313.

25 Tang, C., et al., 'The relationships between high-fat diet and metabolic dysfunction: a narrative review', *Journal of Functional Foods*, advance online publication, 2024, https://doi.org/10.1016/S2212-4292(24)00691-6.

4 Carbohydrates

1 Banfalvi, G., 'Why ribose was selected as the sugar component of nucleic acids' *DNA and Cell Biology* 25(3): 189–96, 2006, https://doi.org/10.1089/dna.2006.25.189.

2 Berg, J. M., et al., *Biochemistry*, 9th ed., W. H. Freeman & Company, 2019.

3 Klein, S., et al., 'Why does obesity cause diabetes?', *Cell Metabolism* 34(1): 11–20, 2022, https://doi.org/10.1016/j.cmet.2021.12.012.

4 National Institute of Nutrition, *Indian Food Composition Tables*, Indian Council of Medical Research, Department of Health Research, Ministry of Health and Family Welfare, Government of India, 2017.

5 Mao, T., et al., 'Effects of dietary fiber on glycemic control and insulin sensitivity in patients with type 2 diabetes: A systematic review and meta-analysis', *Journal of Functional Foods* 82, 104500, 2021, https://doi.org/10.1016/j.jff.2021.104500.

6 Raymond, J. L., and K. Morrow, *Krause and Mahan's Food & the Nutrition Care Process,* 16th ed., Elsevier, 2022.

7 Srilakshmi, B., *Nutrition Science*, 7th ed., New Age International Publishers, 2021.

8 Ibid.

9 Kempner, W., 'Treatment of hypertensive vascular disease with rice diet', *The American Journal of Medicine* 4(4): 545–77, 1948, https://doi.org/10.1016/0002-9343(48)90441-0.

10 James, S.A., 'New low-calorie rice could help cut rising obesity rates', Paper presented at the 249th ACS National Meeting and Exposition, Denver, CO, March 2015.

11 Chapagai, M.K., et al., 'Glycaemic index values and physicochemical properties of five brown rice varieties cooked by different domestic cooking methods', *Functional Foods in Health and Disease* 6(8): 506–18, 2016.

12 Liljeberg, H., and I. Björck, 'Delayed gastric emptying rate may explain improved glycaemia in healthy subjects to a starchy meal with added vinegar', *European Journal of Clinical Nutrition* 52(5): 368–71, 1998, https://doi.org/10.1038/sj.ejcn.1600572.

13 National Institute of Nutrition, *Indian Food Composition Tables*, Indian Council of Medical Research, Department of Health Research, Ministry of Health and Family Welfare, Government of India, 2017.

14 Du, H., et al., 'Fresh fruit consumption and all-cause and cause-specific mortality: findings from the China Kadoorie Biobank', *International Journal of Epidemiology* 46(5): 1444–55, 2017, https://doi.org/10.1093/ije/dyx042.

15 U.S. Department of Agriculture, FoodData Central. (n.d.). *FoodData Central — Food Details for ID 1903944,* https://fdc.nal.usda.gov/food-details/1903944/nutrients

16 National Institute of Nutrition, *Indian Food Composition Tables*, Indian Council of Medical Research, Department of Health

Research, Ministry of Health and Family Welfare, Government of India, 2017.

17 Kawano, Y., et al., 'Microbiota imbalance induced by dietary sugar disrupts immune-mediated protection from metabolic syndrome', *Cell* 185(19): 3501–19.e20, 2022, https://doi.org/10.1016/j.cell.2022.08.005.

18 Polat, C., et al., 'The Relationship Between Nutrition Habits, BMI, Anxiety, and Seborrheic Dermatitis', *Dermatologic Therapy* 38(2), e17781, 2025, https://doi.org/10.1111/dth.17781.

19 National Institute of Nutrition, *Indian Food Composition Tables*, Indian Council of Medical Research, Department of Health Research, Ministry of Health and Family Welfare, Government of India, 2017.

5 What Should We Cook Today?

1 Herpich, C., U. Müller-Werdan, and K. Norman, 'Role of plant-based diets in promoting health and longevity', *Maturitas* 165: 47–51, 2022, https://doi.org/10.1016/j.maturitas.2022.07.003.

2 National Cancer Institute, Cancer trends progress report, U.S. Department of Health and Human Services, National Institutes of Health, April 2025, https://progressreport.cancer.gov.

3 Anjana, R. M., et al., 'Dietary profiles and associated metabolic risk factors in India from the ICMR-INDIAB survey-21', *Nature Medicine* 31(11): 3813–24, 2025, https://doi.org/10.1038/s41591-025-03949-4.

4 Li, L., et al., 'Selected nutrient analyses of fresh, fresh-stored, and frozen fruits and vegetables', *Journal of Food Composition and Analysis* 59: 8–17, 2017.

5 Anand, R., et al., 'Plant-based diet as a precursor to human gut diversity', *Journal of Nutrition*, 2025, https://doi.org/10.1016/j.tjnut.2025.11.020.

6 (Not So) Micro Support Systems

1 Lopresti, Adrian L., 'The Effects of Psychological and Environmental Stress on Micronutrient Concentrations in the

Body: A Review of the Evidence', *Advances in Nutrition* 11(1), 27 August 2019, https://doi.org/10.1093/advances/nmz082.

2 Ministry of Health and Family Welfare, Government of India. 'Compendium of fact sheets: India and 14 States/ UTs (Phase-II)', National Family Health Survey (NFHS-5), 2019–21,https://mohfw.gov.in/sites/default/files/NFHS-5_Phase-II_0.pdf.

3 Roughead, Z.K., C.A. Zito, and J.R. Hunt, 'Initial uptake and absorption of nonheme iron and absorption of heme iron in humans are unaffected by the addition of calcium as cheese to a meal with high iron bioavailability', *American Journal of Clinical Nutrition* 76(2): 419–25, 2002, https://doi.org/10.1093/ajcn/76.2.419.

4 East, P., et al, 'Iron deficiency in infancy and neurocognitive and educational outcomes in young adulthood', *Developmental Psychology* 57(6): 962–75, 2021, https://doi.org/10.1037/dev0001030.

5 Revised Short Summary Report-2024, ICMR-NIN Expert Group on Nutrient Requirements for Indians, Recommended Dietary Allowances (RDA) and Estimated Average Requirements (EAR)-2020.

6 Morck, T.A., S.R. Lynch, and J.D. Cook, 'Inhibition of food iron absorption by coffee', *The American Journal of Clinical Nutrition* 37(3): 416–20, 1983, https://doi.org/10.1093/ajcn/37.3.416.

7 Heffernan, S.M., K. Horner, and S.J. Fairweather-Tait, 'The regulation of dietary iron bioavailability by vitamin C: A systematic review and meta-analysis', *Proceedings of the Nutrition Society* 78(1): 125–35, 2019, https://doi.org/10.1017/S0029665118002846.

8 National Institute of Nutrition, *Indian Food Composition Tables*, Indian Council of Medical Research, Department of Health Research, Ministry of Health and Family Welfare, Government of India, 2017.

9 Revised Short Summary Report-2024, ICMR-NIN Expert Group on Nutrient Requirements for Indians, Recommended

Dietary Allowances (RDA) and Estimated Average Requirements (EAR)-2020.

10 Naciu, A.M., et al., 'Calcium citrate versus calcium carbonate in the management of chronic hypoparathyroidism: A randomized, double blind, crossover clinical trial', *Journal of Bone and Mineral Research* 37(7): 1251–59, 2022, https://doi.org/10.1002/jbmr.4564.

11 Sorensen, M.D., 'Calcium intake and urinary stone disease', *Translational Andrology and Urology* 3(3): 235–40, 2014, https://doi.org/10.3978/j.issn.2223-4683.2014.06.05.

12 Palacios, C., 'The role of nutrients in bone health, from A to Z', *Critical Reviews in Food Science and Nutrition* 46(8): 621–28, 2006, https://doi.org/10.1080/10408390500466174.

13 Barney, A.M., et al., 'Prevalence of Vitamin B12 Deficiency and Its Associated Risk Factors among Pregnant Women of Rural South India: A Community-based Cross-sectional Study', *Indian Journal of Community Medicine* 45(4): 399–404, 2020, https://doi.org/10.4103/ijcm.IJCM_403_19.

14 Revised Short Summary Report-2024, ICMR-NIN Expert Group on Nutrient Requirements for Indians, Recommended Dietary Allowances (RDA) and Estimated Average Requirements (EAR)-2020.

15 Abboud M. 'Vitamin D Supplementation and Sleep: A Systematic Review and Meta-Analysis of Intervention Studies', *Nutrients* 14(5): 1076, 2022, https://doi.org/10.3390/nu14051076.

16 McCarthy, K., et al., 'Association between vitamin D deficiency and the risk of prevalent type 2 diabetes and incident prediabetes: A prospective cohort study using data from The Irish Longitudinal Study on Ageing (TILDA)', *eClinicalMedicine* 53, 101654, 2022, https://doi.org/10.1016/j.eclinm.2022.101654.

17 Revised Short Summary Report-2024, ICMR-NIN Expert Group on Nutrient Requirements for Indians, Recommended Dietary Allowances (RDA) and Estimated Average Requirements (EAR)-2020.

18 Revised Short Summary Report-2024, ICMR-NIN Expert Group on Nutrient Requirements for Indians, Recommended Dietary Allowances (RDA) and Estimated Average Requirements (EAR)-2020.

19 Arjmandfard, D., et al., 'Effects of apple cider vinegar on glycemic control and insulin sensitivity in patients with type 2 diabetes: A GRADE-assessed systematic review and dose-response meta-analysis of controlled clinical trials', *Frontiers in Nutrition* 12, 1528383, 2025, https://doi.org/10.3389/fnut.2025.1528383.

20 AbuMweis, S., et al., 'The ratio of eicosapentaenoic acid to docosahexaenoic acid as a modulator for the cardio-metabolic effects of omega-3 supplements: A meta-regression of randomized clinical trials', *Complementary Therapies in Medicine* 57, 102662, 2021, https://doi.org/10.1016/j.ctim.2021.102662.

21 Wankhede, S., et al., 'Examining the effect of Withania somnifera supplementation on muscle strength and recovery: a randomized controlled trial', *Journal of the International Society of Sports Nutrition 12*(1): 43, 2015, https://doi.org/10.1186/s12970-015-0104-9.

22 Bonilla, D.A., et al., 'Effects of Ashwagandha (Withania somnifera) on Physical Performance: Systematic Review and Bayesian Meta-Analysis', *Journal of Functional Morphology and Kinesiology* 6(1): 20, 2021, https://doi.org/10.3390/jfmk6010020.

23 Zhu, Bingqian, et al., 'Effects of Sleep Restriction on Metabolism-Related Parameters in Healthy Adults: A Comprehensive Review and Meta-Analysis of Randomized Controlled Trials', *Sleep Medicine Reviews* 45: 18–30, June 2019, https://doi.org/10.1016/j.smrv.2019.02.002.

24 Wright, K. P., Jr., et al., 'Influence of sleep deprivation and circadian misalignment on cortisol, inflammatory markers, and cytokine balance', *Brain, Behavior, and Immunity* 47: 24–34, 2015, https://doi.org/10.1016/j.bbi.2015.03.004.

25 Wang, Z., et al., 'Gut microbiota modulates the inflammatory response and cognitive impairment induced by sleep

deprivation', Molecular psychiatry 26(11): 6277–92, 2021, https://doi.org/10.1038/s41380-021-01113-1.

26 Syeda, U.S., et al., 'The importance of exercise for glycemic control in type 2 diabetes', *American Journal of Medicine Open* 9, 100031, 2023, https://doi.org/10.1016/j.ajmo.2023.100031.

27 Kelley, G.A., K.S. Kelley, and Z.V. Tran, 'Resistance training and bone mineral density in women: A meta-analysis of controlled trials', *American Journal of Physical Medicine & Rehabilitation* 80(1): 65–77, 2001, https://doi.org/10.1097/00002060-200101000-00017.

28 Stookey, J.J., 'Negative, null and beneficial effects of drinking water on energy intake, energy expenditure, fat oxidation and weight change in randomized trials: A qualitative review', *Nutrients* 8(1): 19, 2016, https://doi.org/10.3390/nu8010019.

29 Allen, M.D., et al., 'Suboptimal hydration remodels metabolism, promotes degenerative diseases, and shortens life', *JCI Insight* 4(17), e130949, 2019, https://doi.org/10.1172/jci.insight.130949.

30 Kashi, D.S., et al., 'Habitual fluid intake and hydration status influence cortisol reactivity to acute psychosocial stress', *Journal of Applied Physiology*, 2025, https://doi.org/10.1152/japplphysiol.00408.2025.

7 The Anti-Inflammatory Diet

1 International Diabetes Federation, *Diabetes facts and figures*, 2025, https://idf.org/about-diabetes/diabetes-facts-figures/ idf.org.

2 WHO, 'Diabetes – India', 2025, https://www.who.int/india/diabetes.

3 Asian Heart Institute, *Blood sugar level chart by age*, https://asianheartinstitute.org/blog/blood-sugar-level-chart-by-age/.

4 Ahmed, B., R. Sultana, and M.W. Greene, 'Adipose tissue and insulin resistance in obese', *Biomedicine & Pharmacotherapy* 137, Article 111315, 2021, https://doi.org/10.1016/j.biopha.2021.111315.

8 How to Eat

1 Garcidueñas-Fimbres, T.E., 'Associations between eating speed, diet quality, adiposity, and cardiometabolic risk factors',

The Journal of Pediatrics 252: 31–39.e1, 2023, https://doi.org/10.1016/j.jpeds.2022.09.006.

2 Simsek, Y., U.S. Topaloğlu, and O.S. Dizdar, 'High-fructose corn syrup effects on metabolic parameters and malignancy', *Journal of Diabetology* 12(3): 246–251, 2021, https://journals.lww.com/jodb/fulltext/2021/12030/high_fructose_corn_syrup_effects_on_metabolic.2.aspx.

3 Sigala, D. M., et al., 'The Dose-Response Effects of Consuming High Fructose Corn Syrup-Sweetened Beverages on Hepatic Lipid Content and Insulin Sensitivity in Young Adults', Nutrients 14(8): 1648, 2022, https://doi.org/10.3390/nu14081648.

4 Firdous, S., et al., 'Effect of storage temperature and time on the vitamin C contents of selected fruits and vegetables: Vitamin C in fruits and vegetable', *Biological Sciences - PJSIR* 53(4): 218–22, 2010, https://www.biostaging.pjsir.org/index.php/biological-sciences/article/view/462.

5 Clear, J., *Atomic habits: An easy and proven way to build good habits and break bad ones,* Avery, 2018.

9 'Fad Diets', Different Names, Same Principle: Eat Less

1 Oddbjørn, Skartun, et al., 'Symptoms during initiation of a ketogenic diet: a scoping review of occurrence rates, mechanisms and relief strategies', *Frontiers in Nutrition* 12, 2025, https://doi.org/10.3389/fnut.2025.1538266.

About the Author

Amita Gadre is a clinical nutritionist, with over two decades of experience transforming how people understand food, health and sustainable eating. She holds amaster's degree in nutrition and a master's degree in public health from the Tata Institute of Social Sciences, Mumbai, and was awarded a gold medal for academic excellence in nutrition by M.S. University of Baroda. Based in Pune, Amita's clinical practice has reached thousands of clients globally, specialising in lifestyle-related disorders including obesity, diabetes, PCOS, hypothyroidism, hypertension, heart disease, gut health and autoimmune disorders. Her approach is rooted in a simple yet powerful philosophy: all foods are good and can be eaten by everyone; the key lies in understanding how each food functions in the body. Amita's work ethic is equally straightforward: if she wouldn't recommend something to her family, she wouldn't recommend it to her clients.

Want to Learn More?

YouTube
@NutritionistAmita
youtube.com/@NutritionistAmita

Instagram
@amitagadre
instagram.com/amitagadre

E-mail: amita@amitagadre.com